ON THE EPISTEMOLOGY OF THE SENSES IN EARLY CHINESE THOUGHT

The Society for Asian and Comparative Philosophy Monograph Series was started in 1974. Works are published in the series that deal with any area of Asian philosophy, or any other field of philosophy examined from a comparative perspective. The aim of the series is to make available scholarly works that exceed article length, but may be too specialized for the general reading public, and to make these works available in inexpensive editions without sacrificing the orthography of non-Western languages.

MONOGRAPH NO. 19
SOCIETY FOR ASIAN AND COMPARATIVE PHILOSOPHY

ON THE EPISTEMOLOGY OF THE SENSES IN EARLY CHINESE THOUGHT

Jane Geaney

University of Hawai'i Press, Honolulu

Printed in the United States of America

07 06 05 04 03 02 6 5 4 3 2 1

ISBN 0–8248–2557–8
A record of the Cataloging-in-Publication data
can be found at the Library of Congress Website:
http://catalog.loc.gov/

Camera-ready copy for this book was prepared by the author.

University of Hawai'i Press books are printed on acid-free
paper and meet the guidelines for permanence and
durability of the Council on Library Resources.

Printed by Versa Press, Inc.

Contents

Acknowledgments

My study of the early Chinese view of sense discrimination began with dissertation research at the University of Chicago. The early stages of the work profited greatly from careful critical readings by Anthony Yu, Chad Hansen, and Paul Griffiths. The work also profited immensely from the advice and encouragement of Henry Rosemont Jr. I have benefited more from these colleagues' insights than I can adequately acknowledge.

I am thankful to a variety of people who generously helped with the completion of the final draft, especially Lam Ling Hon, for his painstaking attention to the Chinese quotations, Sharon Brinkman for her careful copy editing, George Hardy for repeatedly adjusting the workings of my computer, and Keith Leber for kind and efficient editorial advice. In addition, I would like to thank the anonymous readers from the University of Hawai'i Press. I am also grateful to Dan Robins and Chris Fraser for many fruitful discussions on questions of translation and interpretation. Although I tried to incorporate improvements suggested by these people, the mistakes that remain are soley my responsibility.

Unless otherwise noted, the translations contained herein are my own. Nevertheless, I am inevitably indebted to the following translations, which are doubtlessly reflected in my own: A. C. Graham's *Ch'uang-tzu: the Inner Chapters* (London: George Allen & Unwin, 1981); James Legge's *The Works of Mencius* (Oxford: Clarendon Press, 1895. Reprint, New York: Dover Publications, 1970); W. K. Liao's *The Complete Works of Han Fei Tzu* (London: A. Probsthain, 1935–59); John Knoblock's *Xunzi:A Translation and Study of the Complete Works* (Stanford: Stanford University Press, 1994); Burton Watson's *Hsun-tzu:Basic Writings* (New York: Columbia University Press, 1963); Y. P. Mei's *The Ethical and Political Works of Mo Tse* (London: A. Probsthain, 1929); D. C. Lau's *Mencius* (Baltimore: Penguin Books, 1970) and

Lao Tzu: Tao Te Ching (Harmondsworth, UK: Penguin Books, 1963); and Robert Henricks' *Lao-Tzu Te-Tao Ching: A New Translation Based on the Recently Discovered Ma-Wang-tui Texts* (New York: Ballantine Books, 1989). (I use the *Mawangdui* edition of the *Laozi*, following Henricks in providing the reader with the more familiar *Wang Bi* chapter numbers. Occasionally, in cases where software incapacities or matters of interest make the *Wang Bi* edition more appropriate, I use that edition and note the change.)

I am thankful to the University of Richmond for its generous support in the preparation and publication of this book.

Introduction

This monograph is about sense discrimination in the classical period of Chinese thought.[1] It focuses on the ordinary functions of the human senses, as presented in philosophical texts of the Warring States era (roughly dating from the fifth to third century B.C.E.). As the title suggests, the main senses under consideration are hearing and sight, particularly in relation to the function of the heartmind.[2] A culture's understanding of the physical senses may reveal implicit features of its world view. With that in mind, this work attempts to identify the views on sense discrimination in these texts and subsequently tries to determine what such views imply about the construction of reality in Warring States thought.

This work may have significance for a controversial topic. The results of this analysis seem to corroborate a particular interpretation of early Chinese cosmology—one that views it as distinctive and as having great value.[3] Many features of early Chinese cosmology have been used to argue for its distinctiveness. In this Introduction, I will focus on two of them: its holism and its appreciation of change. The distinctiveness of these features may be highlighted by means of a contrast to the history of western metaphysics.[4] I will outline that contrast in order to explain how my analysis may be used to advance the argument for the distinctiveness of early Chinese cosmology. Then I will describe how the view of sense discrimination in Warring States China supports the contention that early Chinese cosmology is indeed holistic and rooted in change.

Warring States China

A brief historical overview may help situate the texts used in this study. This work is based on the classics of Chinese philosophy, written during what is known as the Warring States period (480–

221 B.C.E.). The Warring States refers to a succession of civil wars among competing territorial states, which took place as a result of the disintegration of the Zhou Dynasty (ca. 1050–256 B.C.E.). The Warring States period ended with the unification of the empire under the Qin, 221–206 B.C.E. Both before and during the Warring States period, a variety of important changes occurred. Within this period, there were significant changes in standards of living: the use of iron developed, especially in agricultural use, and farming replaced hunting as the primary means of sustenance. At the political level, something like a feudal system, based on a hereditary nobility, was replaced by a proliferation of small competing political units, in which power was concentrated in the hands of local monarchs. Through direct taxation on land controlled by the military and hereditary elite, the monarchs effectively eliminated the earlier manorial management system. The result was an increase in social mobility in the form of an opportunity for official court appointments not based on kin relations. In this context, a lower order of artisans emerged and vied for jobs at court. The competition among the states themselves also helped foster an environment in which capable individuals could take on roles that were previously hereditary.

These developments contributed to the rise of a cultural elite that interpreted social ideals. This cultural elite passed on their instruction through disciples, who normally paid a token fee for instruction. Those who were educated could sell their services to territorial states as specialists in things like ritual or even warfare. They often traveled from state to state, in search of an audience for their recommendations regarding social reform. Certain territorial states in particular "collected" some of the most sought-after scholars, giving them titles and stipends, in an effort to enhance their state's reputation. In this role, scholars might have had some small effect on matters of state. More significantly, some of these scholars' words were gathered and written down, forming the texts that are now referred to as classical Chinese philosophy.

Texts

As a particular tradition was passed down from master to disciples, one might speak of "schools of thought" developing in Warring States China.[5] The texts discussed here are later considered to belong to three schools: Confucianism, Mohism, and Daoism. However, because organizing texts into schools of thought was not significant in the Warring States period, it is best not to think of these texts in such terms.[6]

Given modern developments in the field of sinology, it is no longer possible simply to treat Warring States texts as the products of individual authors.[7] Thus, the six texts drawn from here should not be taken as authored by Confucius (d. 479 B.C.E.), Mozi (ca. 480–390 B.C.E.), Mencius (ca. 382–300 B.C.E.), Zhuangzi (ca. 365–280 B.C.E.), Xunzi (ca. 310–215 B.C.E.), or Laozi (dates unknown). Rather, it is probably safest to assume that all of these texts are compilations by a number of authors (of more or less similar persuasion) written over extended periods of time. In other words, we should probably think of these books as *layers* of texts.

Nevertheless, the multilayered nature of these texts need not undermine the main arguments proffered here. The claims I make should be taken as either claims about the philosophical texts of the Warring States period in general or claims about tendencies specifically located within one or another of these texts. (While the latter type of claim involves positing some minimal amount of consistency in the philosophical position represented in a given text, it by no means requires that the texts be the product of single authors.)[8] At this point in the development of sinology, it does not seem possible to do more than make tentative general claims about the view of sense discrimination within the period and within the individual texts. There is barely enough information about sense discrimination in these texts to support even that goal. Given the dearth of data, it is not yet possible to identify nuanced changes in the function of sense discrimination terminology over the course of the Warring States period. If such a thing can ever occur, it must wait until sinology arrives at a greater state of confidence and precision regarding the dating of the layers in these texts. In the meantime, studies like this one may be of use in depicting a particular aspect of the historical period as a whole or trends in individual texts.

There is a reason why this analysis of sense discrimination focuses on philosophical texts, from among the dozens of received texts of the Warring States period. The texts I have chosen are philosophical in a sense that does not necessarily accord with the standards of modern western philosophy. That is, they are philosophical insofar as they employ arguments that have "depth and intricate implicit structure" to engage the subject of ethical and political reform.[9] Because of the deep structure of the arguments in these texts, focusing on them presents a double opportunity. It allows me not only to suggest the current predominant view of sense discrimination, but also to test that hypothesis. In other words, after establishing what I take to be the overarching view of sense discrimination from these texts as a whole, I can also use the individual texts to check the validity of my thesis, by showing how the overarching view functions differently in the deep structure of competing arguments.

The main body of the work describes the predominant view of sense discrimination. The first chapter introduces some general ideas about the senses as a group. The second and third chapters attempt to explain the significance of hearing and sight, as well as their relation to the heartmind. The fourth chapter develops the discussion in relation to a polarity that is particularly important in determining how these texts represent a world view. Finally, the last chapter aims to establish the validity of what I identify as the overarching view of the senses by providing some examples of how that view is put to different uses. The final chapter describes how the shared view of sense discrimination actually functions to support different philosophical positions represented in different texts.

Contrasting Metaphysics

In a work of this sort, comparison and contrast are unavoidable. My ability to understand sense discrimination in the Warring States depends in crucial ways on how I see it in relation to my own tradition. Throughout the work, I explicitly use elements of the tradition more familiar to me to explain what I think is noteworthy about the views represented in the Warring States texts. I presume similarity in the process of selecting the items I think can be compared.[10] But of course I also presume difference, because there is no sense in comparing things that are identical.[11] In my attention to difference, I do not mean to fall into the Orientalist trap of implying that Warring States thought is merely remarkable for its contrast to "the West." As far as possible, this study endeavors to present the intricacies and internal dynamics of Warring States views on its own terms. I hope my determination to do that conveys my conviction that Warring States China has a subjectivity of its own. Still, the best justification for the legitimacy of the comparative elements in this work may be its results. As Ben-ami Sharfstein puts it,

> The question is not whether the differences exist, because they do, but what we should make of them; and the answer often lies in the conscious or unconscious decision to pay no attention to the context, or, more accurately, to make use of only the criteria that fit our need at the time, that is, to intuit or hypothesize or discover the context that is most pertinent to our need.[12]

To that extent, the value of this work may depend on whether I can put these things I have compared into a meaningful context. Especially for non-sinologists, that comparative context may be the most important implication of this study.

The History of Western Metaphysics

The search to identify a permanent substrate of reality was a shared *problematique* in ancient Greek philosophy. The ancient Greeks considered a variety of candidates for this role. For instance, Thales (c. 640–546 B.C.E.) contended that everything was composed of water; Anaximenes (c. 611–547 B.C.E.) argued for the primacy of air. When single elements seemed insufficient, other thinkers proposed combinations, like earth and water, or earth, air, fire, and water.[13] Even Heraclitus (c. 500 B.C.E.), famous for the claim that "everything is becoming," still posited something—fire—as a fundamental eternal substance. Starting with Pythagoras (fl. 540–510 B.C.E.) and his theories of numbers, determining the permanent substrate could also capitalize on the notion of a super-sensible, intelligible world. Hence, in spite of his mistrust of sense perception, Plato (c. 428–348 B.C.E.) could find solace in the clarity with which the intellect knows things like the super-sensible form of the Good. Likewise, Aristotle's (384–322 B.C.E.) confidence lay in a purely formal and unchanging God and the idea that, as matter decreased in proportion to form, things became increasingly stable and knowable. The sensory world of flux and becoming could be transcended in favor of a permanent and eternal foundation. Thus, in various ways, the Greeks managed to identify the permanent foundation of reality.

Underlying their project was the belief that the eternal alone is real. The idea is expressed in its most extreme form by the Eleatic school, which denied the reality of change. Parmenides (fl. 5th cent. B.C.E.) argued that there is no such thing as change, and Zeno (fl. 5th cent. B.C.E.) defended this with various arguments against motion.

The critique of the heritage of this conviction is well known. As Jacques Derrida describes it, the subsequent history of metaphysics perpetuates a particular contradiction.[14] It constructs its notion of presence on the basis of a metaphor of perceptual presence—the moment, or "now." But the now itself is a form of absence, because it is defined by what it is not (the past and the future). If reality is understood on the basis of being present in the moment, then it must in some way be absent. According to Derrida, this language of presence spawns a string of metaphysical oppositions, like intelligible and sensible, soul and body, that are always haunted by the absence of full-presence. Thus, regarding the history of western metaphysics, he says,

> Its matrix...is the determination of Being as presence in all senses of this word. It could be shown that all the names related to fundamentals, to principles, or to the center have always designated an invariable presence *eidos*, *arche*, *telos*, *energeia*, *ousia* (essence, existence, substance, subject), *aletheia*, transcendentality, conscious-ness, God, man, and so forth.[15]

Derrida surveys the later history of western metaphysics, noting how such names for fundamentals continue to designate invariable presence. He identifies "Being as full-presence" as the foundation for the Cartesian cogito. He also finds appeals to a similar grounding in Kant (in the transcendental unity of apperception, which is the noumenon beyond the flux). He uncovers it as well in Hegel's use of self-consciousness. (This condition of all consciousness, Derrida argues, depends on a notion of Being as pure presence.) Likewise, Derrida contends that, in spite of Heidegger's desire to think presence differently than the Greeks, he too presumes that something that *is* must be identical to itself.

All of this, Derrida argues, inherits the Greek conception of eternal self-presence, which is rooted in a metaphor tainted with absence. The language Derrida uses to express this absence is *differance*—difference and deferment. But for the purpose of comparison to early Chinese metaphysics,[16] this might be phrased in terms of change. At the risk of oversimplifying, Derrida's point could be taken as saying that the history of metaphysics succeeds only by repressing change—because change is the difference between the past, the present, and the future. The Greek denial of change (a denial frequently associated with a rejection of the senses) contributed a persistent problem to the history of western metaphysics. According to one interpretation of early Chinese metaphysics, this is a problem that the Chinese of the time did not share.

Metaphysics in Warring States China

The search for something permanent is one of the deepest of the instincts leading men to philosophy.
—Bertrand Russell[17]

At least according to some sinologists, Russell might have found Chinese thinkers to be lacking in a basic philosophical instinct. By contrast to the Greeks, the Warring States Chinese showed no apparent interest in identifying a permanent substrate of reality. Their cosmos was continuous and holistic (in the sense that the parts had to be understood in relation to the whole). It was also subject to a continual process of change.[18] Its philosophers sought only order (rather than Russell's permanence), and the cosmology merely presented a variety of forms of constancy amidst change.

Holism and change are only part of what has been called the "organismic" nature of the early Chinese cosmos.[19] Many additional signs of early Chinese organicism have been highlighted by sinologists. As Donald Munro points out, the application of the term organismic to early China dates back to the work of Joseph Needham, for whom organicism meant, among other things, having developmental patterns like an organism.[20] The idea of organicism is taken up by Frederick Mote, who argues that organicism is evident in the dearth of early Chinese creation myths. Like an organism, he argues, the early Chinese cosmos is not presented as something created *ex nihilo*. Instead, he contends, it is a spontaneous self-generating process.[21] Although Tu Weiming disagrees with Mote's claim about the absence of creation myths, he views early Chinese creation myths as still conforming to the framework of organicism. Tu identifies this framework as having three features: continuity, wholeness, and dynamism.[22] The notion that organicism means continuity is elaborated by Kwang-chih Chang. Chang understands the early Chinese cosmos to be organismic in the sense that it posits no rupture between humanity and its natural resources. Chang's interpretation of organicism suggests (although it does not say so explicitly) that even the nature/culture divide was not fundamental to the formation of early Chinese thought.[23] While all of these understandings of organicism may be valid, in this Introduction I will focus only on holism and change. My purpose will be to show that these two organismic features are also characteristic of the view of sense discrimination in Warring States philosophical texts.

Determining the nature of Warring States cosmology is difficult, because it is neither as overt nor as systematized as it later becomes. When cosmological speculation is fully synthesized (perhaps as early as the end of the Warring States, but certainly by the first century B.C.E.), the cosmos is seen as being composed of *qi* 氣, which appears in two main aspects: as *yinqi* 陰氣 and *yangqi* 陽氣. *Qi* is sometimes rendered "energy/matter," or "psycho-physical stuff"—both translations emphasizing that, although it is material, it resembles energy in being volatile. *Qi* is also connected to breath and wind, but it is sometimes rendered as "vapor" to distinguish it from "air," which is an element (and hence a candidate for a permanent substrate of reality). Unlike an element, *qi* is context dependent. *Yinqi* and *yangqi*, the two main aspects of *qi*, indicate dark, cold, and passive, on the one hand, and bright, warm, and active on the other. But it is significant that something can be *yin* with regard to one thing and *yang* with regard to another. (In addition to its *yin/yang* aspects, in post–Warring States formulations, *qi* also appears as part of the so-called five phases—wood, fire, soil, metal, and water—which relate to one another as conqueror to conquered.) Thus, even in later systematized cosmologies, *qi* is not an eternal substrate—its form changes according to its context.

In the Warring States period, the cosmology based on *qi* was not yet fully systematized in this way. In the philosophical texts, many instances of the character *qi* refer to human *qi* (and, to a lesser extent, animal *qi*). There are also some rarer references to atmospheric *qi*. For instance, there are cases of cloud *qi* (*Zhuangzi* 1/29), heaven and earth's *qi* (*Zhuangzi* 6/68), and night *qi* (*Mencius* 6A8). In one case, *qi* does seem to refer to a fundamental constituent of things. The *Xunzi* notes,

> 水火有氣而無生
> Water and fire have *qi* but do not have life.
> (*Xunzi* 9/69)

However, as of the fourth century B.C.E., the term *qi* did not connote the single basic component of all things. This is apparent in the *Lunyu* 16/7 reference to "blood and *qi*," which suggests that blood did not consist of *qi*. We must be careful then, not to read later cosmological systems back into the Warring States use of *qi*. In Warring States texts, *qi* is an important feature of the cosmos, but it does not have the singular position it later gains. In any case, it is not, in the Warring States or later, a permanent substrate of reality.

The cosmology of the Warring States period is holistic in the sense that all parts are interrelated within the functioning of the whole. Warring States astronomy and calendrics convey a conception of heaven and earth as macrocosm, to which human life should be microcosmically synchronized.[24] With the help of astrology, the Warring States period witnessed the creation of a calendric system that formed a blueprint for the king's behavior by mimicking the regularity of the stars. The *Yi Jing* (*Book of*

Changes) presents similar clues as to the implicit holism in Warring States cosmology. In the *Yi*, one also finds a strong tendency to relate human affairs to natural affairs. Moreover, its hexagrams and line statements indicate inter–dependent relations between important pairs in the cosmos, such as heaven and earth and male and female.[25] Archaeological evidence also points to holistic tendencies in early Chinese cosmology. Mortuary customs from as early as the Shang Dynasty (approximately 1570–1050 B.C.E.) indicate a belief that material goods, such as servants and chariots, would continue to confirm one's status in the afterlife.[26] In a sense, there is nothing "outside of the world," or "other worldly" in this type of afterlife. Oracle bone inscriptions suggest a belief that recently dead ancestors linger close enough to their descendants to be propitiated by sacrificial offerings. With the passage of time, the ancestors show less involvement with the living and presumably become increasingly tenuous, before dissipating entirely. In this holistic picture, heaven and earth, and everything in between, are part of a self-contained continuous creation in which there is no external creative agent and no drastic rupture between creator and created.

Because there is nothing outside the world, Warring States Chinese cosmology cannot help but reconcile itself to changes. As the title of the *Yi Jing* indicates, change is fundamental to the early Chinese cosmos. The *Yi* is a book about change, and within it, even the associations attached to specific images alter according to their context.[27] The creation of astronomical and calendrical systems also depended upon change, that is, they depended upon the ordered celestial regularities associated with the seasons, which set the standards for proper human conduct. Moreover, the transition undergone by deceased ancestors—becoming increasingly detached from social affairs—also represents an afterlife that is not static or atemporal. Rather, the dead ancestor continues to be part of an inevitable dynamic of change.

Like the conception of great cosmic powers, the conception of ordinary people in the Warring States is also holistic. As is frequently noted, the same character (*xin* 心 heartmind) denotes the source of both emoting and thinking. Thus the human person is not broken down into separate reasoning and emoting capacities. The person is also not divided into one immutable soul and an impermanent body. Instead, there are many souls, which separate and disperse after death.[28]

Holism is also apparent in the emphasis on the value of society. From periods prior to and including the Warring States, artistic representations of humans favor depictions of anonymous people working collectively, rather than individual well-known heroes.[29] These collective social relations are also indicated by the Neolithic and Shang practices of burying accompaniers-in-death.[30] Although the practice may have died out by the Warring States, its earlier existence represents a reminder that the bonds uniting persons go beyond even the boundaries of death.

In addition to being holistic, the understanding of the human person also reflects the centrality of change. One of the medical conceptions in the Warring States period identifies health with change.[31] In this conception, the free movement of blood and *qi* in the body's "vessels" guarantees the body's health. Hence, stagnation is the cause of illness. Insofar as freedom of movement was necessary for sustaining the body, a sick person was treated by encouraging a holistic internal motion. Thus, like the cosmos, the ancestors, and the ruler, the composition of the human person was holistic and rooted in change.

In sum, early Chinese cosmology appears to be organismic in its emphasis on holism and change. Perhaps as a result of these organismic features, early Chinese cosmology did not create a metaphysics of presence. This is not to say that early Chinese cosmology is alone in managing this feat, or that early Chinese thought did not create its own set of baneful philosophical problems. However, at least in light of this contrast, early Chinese cosmology seems to have some distinctive value.

Organismic Cosmology and Sense Discrimination

In order to briefly describe the connection between organismic cosmology and the view of sense discrimination I find in these texts, I will, once again, focus on holism and change.

Holism

The presentation of sense discrimination in these texts supports a holistic conception of the human person:

(1) There is no sign of the view that sense discrimination must be transcended in favor of a super-sensible form of knowing.

(2) Sense discrimination itself is characterized by holism, insofar as sensing is integrated into the world. The senses' discriminations are a system constituted by contrasts. The senses discriminate among these contrasts, rather than making contact with brute uninterpreted sense data. Hence, there is nothing in the process of sense discrimination that is pure and untouched by human signification. In other words, there is nothing to mediate and alienate the senses from the world. (For instance, in discriminating between sounds, there are no bare, uninterpreted sound data. Before the ears even hear—which is to say, while they are listening—they establish a continuous interpretive contact. The effort of listening itself channels what is being listened to, framing it within a range of human significance.)

(3) The heartmind is integrated with the other senses. It behaves like the senses and seems to be considered a sense function. It is not distinguished from the other senses in its ability to know its discriminations. Moreover, although it does have a special knowledge capacity (for verifying the operations of seeing and hearing), it does not do so from a position of detachment from the body.

(4) In contrast to the role of vision in Platonic and Cartesian models of knowing, vision is not privileged in this scheme. (Hearing is not privileged either.)[32] The ears and eyes, while performing a more important function than the other senses, maintain a parallel relation with one another. This is not a pseudo-equivalence, veiling a superior term's mastery over an inferior term. Each of the two senses is valued for its strong points and criticized for its weak points. Trust and verification of knowledge requires the participation of both.

Change

No element of sense discrimination escapes change or has contact with a realm outside of change:

(1) The heartmind's pondering is likened to moving eyes in search of a needle. This suggests that the heartmind moves. Ideally, it may be "unmoved"—in the sense of not being led astray by the attractions and repulsions that tug at it. But this sense of being unmoved merely clears the way for the heartmind to respond like a mirror to everything it encounters. (The Warring States metaphor of the mirror indicates responsiveness, rather than re-presentation and detachment.)[33]

(2) Change also plays a significant role in the aural/visual parallels in the text. Change, in the form of action, is the correlate of seeing, just as speech is the correlate of hearing.[34] A form of change is therefore one-half of the equation that constitutes the foundation for trusting people and for verifying knowledge.

(3) The analysis of sense discrimination reveals that there is an element of change implicit in the use of an important character in Warring States philosophical texts. Standard translations of *shi* 實 (as "reality," "substance," or "stuff") do not do justice to the notion of change inherent in the use of the character. Drawing upon the implications of the parallelism between the ears and eyes,

this work calls into question the translations of *shi* in Warring States texts. Traditional understandings of the term *shi* seem to present it as comparable to analytic philosophy's "medium-sized dry goods"—the hard stuff that forms the basis of reference.[35] On the contrary, I argue that the way *shi* functions is best understood as "fruit," due to its organic connotations of growth and development. Although fruit does suggest solidity, my argument is that uses of *shi* have more to do with something brought to completion or fruition, rather than solidity or substance. (After all, in a cosmos where heaven is simply tenuous, while the earth is solid, there is no pressing reason why substance should connote reality.) Translating *shi* as reality, as if that consisted of dry hard goods, leads to a misconception of the notion of reality in Warring States philosophical texts.

This view of sense discrimination fills a gap in our understanding of Warring States thought. Moreover, these elements of holism and change in the view of sense discrimination support the claim that early Chinese cosmology is organismic. They seem to represent one coherent way of understanding the senses from the context of a cosmology in which there is no eternal substrate of reality.

Chapter 1: An Overview of Sense Discrimination

This chapter describes the overarching view of sense discrimination in the philosophical texts of the Warring States period.[1] The individual texts vary in some of their opinions about sense discrimination, but certain shared views about the senses form the backdrop for these variations.[2] In brief, the chapter aims to accomplish two main things: (1) identify the senses and (2) describe their relation to knowledge. The chapter begins by introducing the senses through two focal points of their appearance in these texts: the metaphor of the senses as administrative officials and an image of sense processes carried through the wind. These two focal points highlight some of the complexities and ambiguity of sense discrimination in these texts. They also lay the groundwork for a discussion of the role that the senses play in the acquisition of knowledge, which forms the second half of the chapter.

Identity of the Senses

The Warring States philosophical texts suggest that there are five senses.[3] This number happens to conform to a general tendency to fit things into five-fold schemes.[4] The "fives" include five colors, five tastes, and so on.[5] The *Xunzi* labels the senses as the "five officials" (*wu guan* 五 官), and the texts often list five senses.[6] Moreover, many of the lists of senses look quite a bit like the familiar five–senses model. For instance, *Xunzi* 4/44–45 and *Xunzi* 19/3–5 both list the senses as mouth, nose, eyes, ears, and body; and *Xunzi* 17/11 and 18/116 list the senses as eyes, ears, nose, mouth, and form. *Mencius* 7B24 is similar—it lists mouth, eyes, ears, nose, and limbs. In addition to these lists of five senses, there are also lists of four that sometimes look like the five–senses model with one sense omitted. For example, three cases mention mouth, body, eyes, and ears (not necessarily in that order)—

Mencius 1A7, *Xunzi* 22/80–81, and *Mozi* 32/3–6. With one element replaced, we find eyes, ears, mouth, and form in *Xunzi* 21/14; body, nose, eyes, and ears in *Xunzi* 19/6–8; and ears, eyes, nose, and mouth in *Xunzi* 12/61.[7] In sum, although these lists of sense functions vary and omit items, they are said to number five, and they often include eyes, ears, mouth, nose, and body.

Yet this notion of five senses may be deceptive. Many of the things that appear to be lists of the senses vary remarkably in their number and content.[8] For example, *Mozi* 47/20 seems to list physical organs associated with sensing—mouth, nose, and ears —but fails to mention the eyes and instead includes hands and feet.[9] As in this *Mozi* 47/20 example, the fifth sense is not always the only point of variation. In the *Xunzi*'s lists of the senses, sometimes one or another sense is missing, while the heartmind *and* body (or form) are both included as the fourth and fifth senses respectively.[10] Even more surprisingly, in the *Xunzi*, a possible list of the senses that begins "body, nose, eye, ear," continues with "trust, awe, and peace."[11] Another list mentions eye, ear, mouth, body, form, happiness, and name.[12] Yet another lists eye, ear, mouth, form, and name.[13] The challenge posed by these examples might be evaded by saying that they do not count as lists of the senses. But we might equally well permit these examples to raise doubts about whether any of the lists refer to the senses as we understand them. At the very least, these lists draw attention to the question of what constitutes a sense. Moreover, these lists should be reminders that while there is a compelling reason for the texts to identify the senses as numbering five, there is no firm consensus about the constituents of the senses.

Bureaucracy of the Senses

The metaphor of the senses as officials, and the image linking the senses to the wind (*feng* 風), constitute two of the most striking treatments of sense discrimination in these texts. On the one hand, the metaphor of the senses as officials portrays them as orderly and controlled. Each sense occupies its own office, allowing its desires to be restrained by a superior for the benefit of the "government" of the whole. On the other hand, the role of the wind in sense operations emphasizes a much less controlled environment. The wind turns the senses into a nexus for transformations, both good and bad. With the wind sweeping through them, the senses expose the subject to a potential for radical change. The conflict between these two treatments of the senses does not appear to be resolved in these texts. Perhaps the tensions between these two presentations of the senses are the inevitable result of culling information about the senses from indirect textual references. Or perhaps they are the result of the texts' uncertainty about how the senses function. In either case, an attempt to resolve these tensions might err by forcing coherence on material that is not thoroughly coherent. Hence, I include both descriptions for the sake of accuracy and as a reminder of the confusion in the treatment of the subject of sense operations in these texts.

The primary title for the senses in Warring States philosophical texts identifies them as officials. In addition to the five officials, the *Xunzi* also refers to the senses as the "heavenly officials" (*tian guan* 天 官).[14] The bureaucratic title should not be surprising, because the matter of proper governing is a pressing concern in the Warring States period, evident in all of these texts.[15]

In their behavior as official, each sense is an office with its own area of concern. Many lists articulate the specific role of each function, insisting that they are not identical. For instance, the *Xunzi* emphasizes the specialization of each sense structure:

> 耳目鼻口之不可以相借官
> Ear, eye, nose, and mouth cannot trade offices.
> (*Xunzi* 12/61)

The *Xunzi* and the *Mencius* also emphasize that the officials are ruled by the heartmind.[16] The *Xunzi* says,

> 耳目鼻口形能各有接
> 而不相能也夫是之謂天官
> 心居中虛以治五官
> 夫是之謂天君
>
> Ear, eye, nose, mouth, and form, each has its own contacts [lit. "receptions" or "meetings"] and does not do things for the others. Now, these are called the heavenly officials. The heartmind dwells in the central cavity and governs the five officials. Now, this is called the heavenly ruler.
> (*Xunzi* 17/11–12)

Similarly, *Mencius* 6A5, which also attributes 'offices' to the senses, indicates that the heartmind's job is superior. Hence, just as officials function like senses, the senses behave like officials under the control of a ruler.

The general opinion—expressed rather clearly in the *Xunzi*, the *Mencius*, and the *Mozi*—is that, because of their wayward desires, the senses make better officials than rulers. The senses instigate their own desires. Rather than attributing the desires to a person, or to the heartmind (the ruler of the senses), the *Xunzi* speaks as if the ears themselves desire sound and the eyes themselves desire appearances.[17]

> 若夫目好色耳好聲口好味
> 心好利骨體膚理好愉佚
> 是皆生於人之情性者也
>
> The eyes' love of color,[18] the ears' love of sounds, the mouth's love of flavors, the heartmind's love of profit, the bones, flesh and skin-lines' love of pleasure and ease: these are all born of a person's *qing* [condition? disposition?] and nature.
> *Xunzi* 23/25–26

The senses also share the same respective desires, as the *Mencius*, and the *Mozi* point out.[19] The *Xunzi* notes that we are born with these desires and speaks of them as the human *qing* 情 (condition? disposition?), while the *Mencius* speaks of them as human *xing* 性 (nature/what one is born with).[20] Thus, sensory desires appear to be something very fundamental in human beings that interfere with ordering the person.

These shared sense desires pose dangers to the order of the person by disturbing thinking and tending toward excess. Sense desires contact things, and when their desires make contact, thinking is lost. The *Xunzi* says,

> 耳目之欲接則敗其思蚊虻之聲聞則挫其精
> [re: a man sitting in a cave, trying to concentrate] If the desires of the ears and eyes contact [what they desire], then his thoughts will be defeated, and if he hears the buzzing of mosquitoes or flies, his concentration will be damaged.
> (*Xunzi* 21/62)

The *Mencius* says something similar, noting that the heartmind gets what it seeks, but the senses are pulled by things:

> 耳目之官不思而蔽於物
> 物交物則引之而已矣
> 心之官則思思則得之不思則不得也
> Thinking is not the office of the eyes and ears, and they are clouded by things. Things interact with things and pull them astray. That is all. The office of the heartmind is thinking. It thinks and thus it obtains. If it does not think, then it does not obtain.
> (*Mencius* 6A15)

In addition to distracting one's thinking, sense desires are also inherently inclined toward excess. As the *Xunzi* says,

目欲綦色耳欲綦聲
口欲綦味鼻欲綦臭心欲綦佚
The eyes desire the greatest extreme of colors, the ears desire the greatest extreme of sounds, the mouth desires the greatest extreme of tastes, the nose desires the greatest extreme of smells, the heartmind desires the greatest extreme of comfort.
(*Xunzi* 11/46–47)

This tendency toward excess is implicit in the Mozi's condemnation of wicked kings for not checking the "flow" of their ears and eyes.[21] (This notion of flowing seems to derive from their inability to remain within bounds.)

三代之暴王不繆其耳目之淫
不慎其心志之辟
The wicked kings of the Three Dynasties did not control the flowing of their ears and eyes and did not restrain the partialities of their heartmind's aims.[22]
(*Mozi* 36/18)

The distraction and excesses of the sense desires seem barely controllable. In addition to sharing similar desires, the senses share a similar inability to control them.

In sum, the senses are born instigating desires. These desires distract the heartmind from its ability to think and accomplish its aims. They are also dangerously excessive and lead naturally toward inauspicious and immoral extremes. Because their desires are distracting and excessive, the senses must be restrained. This seems to account for why the senses may function only as officials under the control of a ruler, without ever being rulers themselves. With characteristic iconoclasm, the *Zhuangzi* disagrees. It implies that the vassals and concubines of the body might take turns being ruler.[23] But even the *Zhuangzi*'s objection supports the point—if the purpose is order and control, the senses should be officials (*guan*) rather than rulers (*jun*).

Sensing the Wind

The sensory aspects of the wind (*feng* 風) provide a contrasting illustration of how the senses function.[24] Instead of being clearly organized officials with separate offices, sensing the wind hints at subtle, blended forms of sensing. For example, while being carried on the wind, music seems to spontaneously transform through the senses, at the infinitesimal level of *qi* 氣 (vapor) and *de* 德 (charisma/virtue).[25] In addition to this audible sensing, harmonious winds/airs seem to have simultaneous effects on olfactory and gustatory sensing. From this perspective, sense discrimination appears to be a chaotic and unmanageable process.

Oracle inscriptions from the Shang Dynasty (eighteenth through twelfth century B.C.E.) suggest that winds were an object of pressing concern for the ancient Chinese. The evidence indicates that divination rituals were performed to determine all kinds of questions about winds.[26] The importance of wind continued to figure in Warring States philosophical texts. The *Zhuangzi* depicts the movements of the cosmos as a great blowing wind, impelling force in cavities like ears, nostrils, and eye sockets (*Zhuangzi* 2/4–9). The sensory aspects of wind apparent in the Warring States texts may explain some of this concern about winds. Sensing the wind produces automatic transformation. It seems to involve a powerful mix of elements that immediately alter whomever hears or "ingests" it.

Music is the most outstanding thing sensed through contact with the wind. It changes people by affecting their winds/airs. (Like the word "air" in English, the term *feng* 風 also functions to mean the style that is characteristic of a place or a group of people.) The *Xunzi* extols the powers of music to improve such winds:

> 樂者聖人之所樂也
> 而可以善民心其感人深其移風易俗
> Music is the joy of the sages.[27] It can improve people's heartminds. It stimulates people deeply. It influences their wind [*feng*] and changes their customs.
> (*Xunzi* 20/22–23)

The metaphor of people's wind being transformed by music presumes that sound is sensed via its carrier: the wind. It seems that because the style of a group is its wind, the style can be molded by the sounds of music, which are carried on the wind.

At a more intricate level, the power of music can be explained as the transmission of infinitesimal things like *qi* and *de*. Both wind and music are spoken of in terms of *qi*. This is noteworthy, because references to the *qi* of specific things are quite rare in these texts.[28] From the reference to the piping of *qi* in the *Zhuangzi* and the two references to music's *qi* in the *Xunzi*, we can infer that *qi* is more closely associated with wind and music than it is with most things. According to the *Zhuangzi*, wind is the *qi* that the earth exhales while piping its music.[29] If wind is the piped *qi* of earth, then to an extent, *qi*, wind, and music are interchangeable. Moreover, the *Xunzi* refers to music as *qi*, when explaining the powerful effects of the sounds of singing. It says,

> 凡姦聲感人而逆氣應之
> 逆氣成象而亂生焉
> 正聲感人而順氣應之
> 順氣成象而治生焉
> 唱和有應善惡相象
> 故君子慎其所去就也
> When chaotic sounds stimulate a person, the response is an oppositional *qi*. When an oppositional *qi* forms a shape, thereupon disorder is born. When upright sounds stimulate a person, the response is a compliant *qi*. When a compliant *qi* forms a shape, thereupon order is born. The

> singer and the harmonizer have [mutual?] responses. Good and bad take shape correspondingly. Therefore, noble people are careful about their goings and comings.
> (*Xunzi* 20/26–28)

The pattern of stimulation and response, along with the reference to singer and harmonizer implies that music achieves its effect—whether positive or negative—through the power of resonating *qi*.[30] In another reference to the *qi* of music, the *Xunzi* warns that this stimulating resonance must be restrained. (As the passage begins, the *Xunzi* notes that chaos will ensue if people are not free to use the expression of music/joy as their guide.)

> 先王惡其亂也故制雅頌之聲以道之
> 使其聲足以樂而不流
> 使其文足以辨而不諰
> 使其曲直繁省廉肉節奏足以感動人之善心
> 使夫邪汙之氣無由得接焉
> The kings of old hated such chaos. Therefore, they regulated the sounds of the Odes and Hymns in order to guide [*dao*] them [the people]. They caused the sounds to be sufficient for joy, but not flowing. They caused the forms to be sufficient to discriminate, but not restrictive. They caused the intricacy or the directness, the abundance or the scarcity, the modesty or the corporeity of the rhythm and performance to be sufficient to stimulate and move people's good heartminds. They thereby made sure corrupt and impure *qi* could not make contact therein. (*Xunzi* 20/3–4)

The passage's reference to not letting the *qi* of music gain "contact" (*jie* 接) suggests that the resonating *qi* described here is contacting the senses.[31] Thus, this contact with musical *qi* probably indicates contact through the senses.[32] This clarifies what occurs when a people's style (wind) is influenced by music (as in

Xunzi 20/22). Music transforms the wind via the intake of *qi* through the senses. The resonance of the musical *qi* automatically alters the person who senses it, causing an expulsion of similar *qi*. In other words, *qi* is the music that enters the senses as well as the wind that the music causes to emerge from them.

In addition to *qi*, the potency of music also works by means of *de*—something that is accessible to the senses, but as nebulous as *qi*.[33] The *Mencius* notes that *de* can be heard through music.

> 子貢曰見其禮而知其政聞其樂而知其德
> Zigong said, "By viewing his ceremonies we know his administration. By hearing his music, we know his *de*." (*Mencius* 2A2)

De is as light as a hair (*Xunzi* 16/75), but it is often referred to as "ample" or "thick." This is because *de* can accumulate.[34] The accumulation of *de* fills out into visual, and especially aural, forms.[35] The *Mozi* and the *Xunzi* speak repeatedly of the effects of "*de* and tone"—emphasizing the transmission of *de* through sound. In the course of explaining that the ancient kings increased their efficiency by seeking help from others, the *Mozi* suggests that the lips that emit speech are the medium by which *de* is spread:

> 非神也夫唯能使人之耳目助己視聽
> 使人之吻助己言談
> 使人之心助己思慮
> 使人之股肱助己動作
> 助之視聽者眾則其所聞見者遠矣
> 助之言談者眾則其德音之所撫循者博矣
> 助之思慮者眾則其談謀度速得矣
> 助之動作者眾即其舉事速成矣
> [The ancient kings said] "It [their own effectiveness] was not the spirits,[36] but only the ability to use others' ears and eyes to help their own hearing and sight to use others' *lips*

> *to help their own speech and talk*, to use others' heart-minds to help their own thought, to use others' limbs to help their movements and acts." When those who help one's listening and looking are many, then one can hear and see far. When those who help one's *speech and talk* are many, then the soothing and compelling aspects of one's *de and tone* are extensive.[37] When those who help one's thinking and pondering are many, then one's talk, plans and operations can be attained quickly. When those who help one's movements and acts are many, then one's undertakings can be quickly accomplished.
> (*Mozi* 12/65–67, emphasis added)

This claim that *de* is enhanced by the lips of others suggests that *de* functions orally/aurally. Moreover, the association of *de* with tone reinforces the claim in *Mencius* 2A2 that music provides evidence of *de*. A less literal interpretation might take all this to refer to spoken descriptions of virtue. But interpreting *de* at that level of abstraction does not explain why *de* is so often spoken of, rather than seen.[38] Nor does it explain the connection of *de* to music.

The power of music may also be linked to the harmony that produces *de*. *De* and tone are "soothing and compelling" (*Mozi* 12/66 above); they "fill and soothe the hundred clans" (其德音足以填撫百姓, *Xunzi* 12/102).[39] This power to soothe may well derive from the harmony that seems to create *de*. The *Zhuangzi* explains *de* through the concept of cultivating harmony to the point of completion:

> 德者成和之脩也
> *De* is the cultivation of completed harmony.
> (*Zhuangzi* 5/47)

It seems justifiable to take this harmony as referring to music, because the *Zhuangzi* also speaks of the harmony of *de* via a metaphor suggestive of wind (which, as we have just seen, is the carrier of music). The metaphor implies that the harmony that creates *de* is like a wind upon which people can roam:

> 遊心乎德之和
> They let the heartmind roam upon the harmony of *de*.
> (*Zhuangzi* 5/8)

This roaming is suggestive of the wind, because the *Zhuangzi*'s sages tend to roam on wind and/or *qi*. For instance, the *Zhuangzi* chastises the character Liezi, whose riding on wind seems inferior to riding on *qi* (or roaming in the boundless):[40]

> 列子御風而行
> 此雖免乎行猶有所待者也若夫乘天地之正而御六氣之辯以遊無窮者彼且惡乎待哉
> Liezi moved with the wind as his chariot....Although this avoids walking, it still depends on something. But ascending straight through heaven and earth, taking the changes of the six *qi* as one's chariot, and roaming that which has no boundaries—how is that depending on anything?
> (*Zhuangzi* 1/19–21)

This airborne "roaming" links roaming on the harmony of *de* to roaming on wind or *qi*. As the passages discussed above indicate, music is transported on wind or *qi*. Because it travels on wind or *qi*, the harmony of *de* may well be musical, and it may derive its capacity to soothe from its musical tones. If so, it is because wind carries resonant (musical) *qi* and the soothing (musical) harmonies that create *de*. By this means, the wind enters the ears and transforms the person who hears it.

But the powers of wind are not limited to hearing music. At times, wind transforms through being ingested in other ways, and at times its effects overlap with more than one sense. The metaphor in *Zhuangzi* 2/4 (see Chapter 1, footnote 29) of exhaling the *qi* of earth is one example wherein wind and *qi* are exhaled. They can also be inhaled and, in a surprising number of circumstances, affect one's desire for food. For instance, the *Zhuangzi* mentions an inverse relation between depth of breathing and relish of taste. Regarding the true people of old, it says,

> 其食不甘其息深深
> Their eating is not sweet. Their breathing is deeply deep.
> (*Zhuangzi* 6/6)

Similarly, the *Zhuangzi* also describes a "spirit person" (*shenren* 神人), who inhales wind instead of eating:

> 藐姑射之山有神人居焉...
> 不食五穀吸風飲露
> In the mountains of far-off Guyi resides a *shen*-person, who...does not eat the five grains, but inhales the wind and drinks the dew.
> (*Zhuangzi* 1/28–29)

By inhaling (odorless?) wind and (tasteless?) dew, the person is transformed into an airy creature of the mountain heights. Although the quality of the taste/smell is not mentioned in this passage, one can only imagine that, as in *Zhuangzi* 6/6, this inhaling has replaced ordinary food with a rather bland diet.

A similar phenomenon may be operative in the *Lunyu*. Confucius loses his appreciation for food upon being exposed to impressive music:

> 子在齊聞韶三月不知肉味
> When the Master was in Qi, he heard the Shao music—for three months he did not know the taste of meat.
> (*Lunyu* 7/14)

Of course, the main point is that Confucius was completely absorbed in the joy provided by the music. However, the manifestation of his preoccupation is striking. Like the person in *Zhuangzi* 1/29 who inhales wind instead of food, Confucius's ingestion of music seems to counteract his desire for savory food. This may explain why Confucius does not know (the desire for) taste—he is already filled by the winds of music.

Like music in the case of the *Lunyu*, *de* causes a loss of taste in the *Mencius*. Explicating a passage from the *Book of Poetry*, it says a person who is full of *de* is like a person with a full stomach:

> 詩云既醉以酒既飽以德
> 言飽乎仁義也
> 所以不願人之膏粱之味也
> 令聞廣譽施於身所以不願人之文繡也
> The *Book of Poetry* says, "He intoxicates us with his wine. He satiates us with his *de*." That is, he satiates them with humaneness and righteousness, hence they do not desire the taste that people have for fat meat and fine millet. A fine reputation and broad praise are bestowed upon their persons, hence they do not desire people's elegant embroidered garments.
> (*Mencius* 6A7)

Here too *de* is as satisfying as food, and it overwhelms the ordinary desires of taste.

Another passage from the *Mencius* may also suggest transformation via inhaling wind, although "hearing reputation" is the more acceptable translation. *Mencius* 5B1 speaks of people being influenced by the wind of a person of good character. It says,

> 故聞伯夷之風者
> 頑夫廉懦夫有立志

> Therefore, of those who hear/smell[41] the wind of Bo Yi, the obstinate become pure, the weak become erect in their intent.
> (*Mencius* 5B1)

If wind is taken to refer to Bo Yi's reputation, the passage may describe the sound of Bo Yi's good name being transmitted by the wind. But the passage does not mention reputation. Thus, because the wind can be smelled as well as heard, this passage may also be invoking the transformative power of inhaling wind. Hence, in addition to the transformative powers of hearing music, the wind can transform in other ways. Its effects are felt in the senses of smell and taste, as well as hearing.

A loose connection seems to bind these elements carried on the wind—one hears them, exhales or inhales them, and even sometimes has them substitute for oral ingestion. Wind is the carrier of music, whose influence seems to derive from the resonance of *qi* and the harmonies of *de*. In whatever form, however, sensing the wind has powerful transformative effects. These effects account for some of the perceived power of the wind. They also suggest a somewhat unruly potential inherent in the senses, through which the wind operates.

Knowledge and Sense Discrimination

Whether sense discrimination resembles a bureaucracy or a windstorm, the senses indisputably play a role in the acquisition of knowledge. The references to the senses' participation in knowing are often brief or cryptic. However, I will argue that they yield an intelligible portrait of the senses' role in knowing.

Briefly, there are two kinds of knowledge associated with sense discrimination in Warring States philosophical texts: (1) "Sensory knowledge" refers to knowledge of the senses themselves, independent of the heartmind. (2) "Verifying knowledge" refers to knowledge that is constructed by a combination of certain senses and the heartmind. In order to clarify the nature of these two types of sense knowledge, I will compare them with three models of sense knowledge in Western philosophy: sensation, perception, and aspect perception. I will argue that sensation and perception are significantly different from the kinds of knowledge associated with the senses in these texts, but that aspect perception bears some resemblance to them.

Comparative Models of Sense Knowledge

Sensation

Sensation is a model of sense knowledge that arises in the context of a realist versus idealist debate about sense discrimination. Broadly speaking, in that debate, realists argue that the senses have some kind of direct contact with external objects in the world. By contrast, idealists maintain that objects as we know them are significantly constructed by their contact with the mind. Idealists argue that realists underestimate the role of the operations of the mind in the sensory process. Thus, according to idealists, we do not have *direct* contact with external objects.

The model of sensation I describe here derives from a position called representative realism that attempts to bridge the two poles of realism and idealism. For the representative realist, the term "sensation" means the direct, private awareness of sense data. Sense data are content neutral and uninterpreted. For instance, I might have the sensation of seeing a patch of red.[42] If I have that sensation, I may insist that I see the sense data, regardless of whether anyone else sees it or whether there is an actual external object that corresponds to it. Sensation is supposed to indicate what the experience is like "to me" (once again, regardless of what is outside). The knowledge attributed to sensation is infallible: I cannot be wrong about having a sensation that I see a red patch.[43]

Perception

Perception also plays a role in the representative realist model of sense knowledge. Unlike sensation, perception is indirect. It interprets the sense data.[44] Thus, it is supposed to indicate something about the object, as opposed to the red patch that I see. Because the beliefs involved in perception are interpreted, they are potentially fallible. Whereas sensation cannot be wrong about amorphous things like patches of red, perception's interpretation of such data contains the possibility of error—for instance, when it identifies a patch of red as, say, a fire engine.

As this brief sketch of representative realism indicates, sensation and perception refer to two different (often opposed) modes of understanding how knowledge may be acquired by the senses. The knowledge that is possible in sensation involves 'raw data,' no interpretation, and no error. Knowledge in perception is indirect, and beliefs based on perception can be wrong because of the interpretation of raw data.

Aspect Perception

Ludwig Wittgenstein's model of "aspect perception" draws a distinction between "seeing" and "seeing as."[45] The latter refers to seeing "aspects." For instance, seeing an aspect means seeing a face *as* a face and not a flesh color with a certain shape. In looking at a sketch that sometimes seems like a rabbit and sometimes a duck, one sees aspects, when one regards it *as* a rabbit or *as* a duck. Even if we quickly switch back and forth from seeing it as a rabbit to seeing it as a duck, aspect-seeing is characteristically continuous in a particular sense—it is not a disjointed inference drawn from a hypothesis. As Wittgenstein explains, upon viewing a duck/rabbit sketch, we do not say "Oh, if I see this part as an ear and this part as the top, then it looks like a rabbit." Rather, we say, "Now it's a duck! Now it's a rabbit!" In other words, seeing aspects is not a kind of seeing that is followed by thinking and then drawing an inference about what is seen.[46] That is, although it involves treating things *as* something, aspect-perception is not the same as perception (described above). Unlike perception, it is not mediated by an act of interpreting raw data. It is embedded in a context (in which, for instance, knowing rabbits and ducks is taken for granted). This background gives it a spontaneity not characteristic of making hypotheses and drawing inferences.

In spite of its immediateness, aspect perception does not have the infallible certainty of sensation. Unlike sensation, it regards things meaningfully, in the sense that things are perceived *as* something.

Neither perception nor sensation fits the models of sense discrimination in these Warring States texts. The knowledge affiliated with the senses is not sensation, because it is not the private knowledge of sense data. Furthermore, because there is no notion of sense data, the sensory knowledge also does not fit the perception model—wherein the mind interprets the data.

The fact that these models are not appropriate is not surprising, because the idealist/realist debate is not operative in Warring States philosophy. In these Warring States texts, the distinction between things "as they seem to us" and things "as they are in themselves" is not a philosophical problem. Of course, the texts notice cases where one or more of the senses seems unreliable, but they do not proceed to express skepticism about the senses as a whole.[47] They manifest no concern about the senses systematically distorting "things as they are." Thus, ideas about private, immediately known sense data do not appear in these texts. In other words, in keeping with the fact that the texts do not doubt the reliability of the senses as a whole, they also do not need a notion like sense data to allay their doubts.

Although the realist/idealist debate is not evident in Warring States philosophical texts, their epistemological position is not naive realism. It might be called naive, insofar as it is naive not to entertain questions about being systematically deluded by the senses. Yet, by not debating realism versus idealism, the position does not, by default, become the naive realist confidence that colors and sounds are somehow in the surfaces of objects. It treats things like colors and sounds as things in their own right, not as things that *belong* to objects.[48] Moreover, the default position in these texts does not take the stand that colors and sounds simply belong "out there" in the world. Although the texts do not assert that consciousness shapes things like colors and sounds, their default position is not that things exist without any connection to human context. Rather, the epistemological position seems to take for granted the influence of background in sense discrimination. The texts suggest that things are sensed in terms of their connections to a range of similar types of things. This is evident in the *Xunzi*'s selection of the character "discriminate" (*bian* 辨) to indicate what the senses do.[49] Discriminate is also the term the *Xunzi* uses to describe what names do. Thus it is not that the senses are natural and names are conventional—names and the senses are similar. Just as names depend upon a system of differences (one name can only function by means of not being another name), so too any given sense discrimination (such as sweet) gains its identity by not being something else (such as salty or sour). The identity of what is sensed depends in part on relations to other sensed things. Furthermore, the subjects who make sense discriminations are also part of the constitutive relations among things. Rather than bracketing the role of the human beings who sense, in their discussions of sense discrimination the texts emphasize factors like desire and aversion (that is, often the examples of sensing involve desirable and undesirable things). The texts also imply that the very attempt to sense something already entails *regarding* the thing in some way. Thus, if there is such a thing as a range of colors "out there," it would have to be unavailable to even the most basic form of sensing. Moreover, the texts begin their analysis of the senses with the human being in the midst of sensing.[50] Although it is not naive realism, this position is realistic in its confidence that it is possible to have constant standards for sensory and naming discriminations. In these texts, this position contrasts with relativistic perspectivism—a position that maintains that we cannot have constant standards for sensory and naming discriminations, because there is no constant perspective.[51]

In sum, the poles of idealism versus realism do not seem important in Warring States philosophical texts. Whether things, such as colors, are out there or in the sensing subject is not in question. But that does not mean that, by default, the texts imply that colors are merely out there. Instead, a color must be discriminated in terms of a background of other colors and the preferences associated with that form of discrimination.

Sensory Knowledge in Warring States Philosophical Texts

My contention is that there is sensory knowledge in these texts that is independent of the heartmind. This knowledge is mentioned in the *Zhengming* (Rectification of Names) chapter of the *Xunzi*, in a lengthy passage that describes the operations of the senses. It also appears in a number of other passages.

Before presenting the evidence for sensory knowledge, it is necessary to briefly sketch the *Zhengming*'s discussion of sense discrimination. The *Zhengming* introduces the function of the senses in the course of its description of the "causes for sameness and difference." The context of the discussion of the senses is an explanation of how a qualified ruler would go about rectifying names for the purpose of establishing order. A knowledgeable ruler would clarify important distinctions—like those between nobility and baseness and the very difference between sameness and difference itself. The *Zhengming* inquires about what constitutes the causes for sameness and difference and then answers its own question. The answer seems to come in three stages: (1) a description of sameness, (2) a description of difference, and (3) a description of knowledge.

The reference to the senses having knowledge occurs in the third section, along with a more detailed description of something called "verifying knowledge" (in which the heartmind works with certain senses). The *Zhengming* notes a series of conditions required for verifying knowledge. It seems to say that if there is recording without knowing, or verifying without speaking, then the person will not be credited with knowing:[52]

> 然而徵知必將待天官當簿其類
> 然後可也
> 五官簿之而不知心徵之而無説
> 則人莫不然謂之不知
> However, verifying must await the heavenly officials' meeting and recording their kinds in order to be possible. If the five officials record them without knowing, or if the heartmind verifies without speaking,[53] then people will not fail to pronounce it "not knowing."
> (*Xunzi* 22/19–21)

I take it that the agent with the potential to know in the third line refers to the sense officials themselves, rather than the heartmind.

This is not the only passage in the *Xunzi* that seems to attribute knowledge to the senses themselves. In another passage, the *Xunzi* also considers cases in which the senses do *not* know in a way that implies that ordinarily they *do* know. The passage describes cases wherein sensory knowledge is in jeopardy—when principle is treated lightly, when external things are valued, when behavior departs from principle, and when the body is threatened. When the heartmind is distracted in these ways, the *Xunzi* says,

> 口銜芻豢而不知其味
> 耳聽鐘鼓而不知其聲
> 目視黼黻而不知其狀
> 輕煖平簟而體不知其安
> The mouth may be holding fine meats, but it does not know their flavor. The ears may listen to bells and drums, but they do not know their sound. The eyes may see embroidered, ornamented garments, but they do not know

> their form. Though it has cold and warmth, peace and a fine bamboo mat, the body does not know their ease.
> (*Xunzi* 22/80–81; Knoblock trans. modified 3:138)

A passage from the *Mozi* confirms that the senses can be spoken of as knowing. The *Mozi* says (of music, ornament, delicious food, and nice places to live),

> …身知其安口知其甘目知其美耳知其樂也
> …the body knows their comfort, the mouth knows their sweetness, the eyes know their beauty, and the ears know their music.
> (*Mozi* 32/5–6)

Even if this type of knowing might translate more readily as "awareness," the fact is, the texts developed no distinct term for awareness.[54] Hence, the same term for knowing is used both for the senses and for the knowing attributed to the heartmind. To that extent, it is fair to say that the senses *do* know.

If the senses know, then the *Zhengming*'s long description of sense operations should yield some clues about the nature of their knowledge. The *Zhengming*'s description begins with the "cause for sameness":

> 凡同類同情者其天官之意物也同
> 故比方之疑似而通
> 是所以共其約名以相期也
> For anything of the same *lei* [kind] and the same *qing* [condition? disposition?], the heavenly officials' "intentional thing"[55] is the same. Thus, by lining up their [the senses'] areas of doubts and similarities, and making them universal,[56] they [the knowledgeable rulers alluded to earlier?] make public [common?] the respective limits of "fixed names."[57]
> (*Xunzi* 22/16)

This brief comment on the "cause of sameness" culminates with an assertion that sameness builds from public agreement about habits of naming.[58]

It is easy to see how this description of the cause for sameness leads to misinterpretations of the *Xunzi*'s view of sense discrimination. In the first line, the term *qing* 情 has been translated as "essential characteristics."[59] However, in this context, the term *qing* 情 is probably no more philosophically weighty than the term *lei* 類 (kind). Hence, "things of the same kind and condition/disposition" together suggest "generally similar things." This section on the causes for sameness seems to claim that the senses move in similar directions toward similar things, that is, the passage asserts that, regarding things that are generally similar, the heavenly officials will have similar *yiwu* 意 物. The Chinese character *yi* 意 is frequently translated as "idea," which in this context, might give the unfortunate impression of something like representative mental ideas.[60] An immediate reason to reject such an interpretation of the passage is that the *yiwu* belongs to the sense officials, not the heartmind. Furthermore, translating *yi* 意 as "representation" or "idea" is misleading, because of the visual connotations of these terms in much of the Western philosophical tradition.[61] Emphasis on the visual is belied by the aural element in the constitution of this character—"tone" *yin* 音, over the "heartmind" *xin* 心. Finally, such an interpretation is also unlikely because *yi* is not internal.

Yi 意 is better translated as "intent"—in the sense of something external and manifest in movement. This is apparent because the *Xunzi* attributes "intentionality" to a dance:

> 舞意天道兼....
> 曷以知舞之意
> 曰目不自見耳不自聞也
> 然而治俯仰詘信進退遲速
> 莫不廉制

> The intent [*yi* 意] of the dance joins with the way of heaven....How can one know the intent of the dance?—The eyes do not themselves see, the ears do not themselves hear,[62] and yet the order of the bowing, raising the head, crouching and stretching out, advancing and retreating, slowing down and speeding up is such that none of it is not modest and controlled.
> (*Xunzi* 20/37–39)

Thus, *yi* is not an internal mental picture at all. As in the orderly movement of the dance, *yi* is a manifest and measurable *tending* or movement. On these grounds, it seems that the senses' *yiwu* (intentional thing) refers to the direction of the senses' movement or inclination in relation to things. Thus, the description of the cause for sameness describes a process whereby the senses share a tendency with regard to similar things—a tendency to move in similar directions toward similar things.[63]

This notion that the senses have an intention or a direction helps explain sensory error and, by extension, sensory knowledge. These texts mention two things that cause the senses to fail to know. *Xunzi* 22/80–81 (see above) describes how the heartmind's preoccupations can distract the senses from knowing what is right in front of them. The implications of this are often noticed, and the passage is taken as saying that the senses' knowledge is like perception—the mind is necessary for the senses to know. However, the presence of other obstructers of sensory knowing—like darkness, distance, and pressure from the hands—suggests a different conclusion.[64] That is, sensory error can be caused by *any* obstruction in the direction toward which it is headed. For instance, the Mencius cites hunger and thirst as such obstructions:

> 飢者甘食渴者甘飲是未得飲食之正也
> 飢渴害之也

> The hungry sweeten [or "find sweetness in"] eating. The thirsty sweeten drinking. This is not obtaining the correctness of eating and drinking. [It is because] hunger and thirst obstruct them.
> (*Mencius* 7A27)

Hence, sensory knowledge depends, not on the heartmind's attention per se, but on freedom from having its directions/intentions obstructed (whether by the heartmind or the hands, or anything else).

Xunzi 21/70 attributes sensory error to the influence of various things on other things. It notes that darkness will make a person confuse a stone for a tiger and that drunkenness will change a person's ability to judge spatial distance. It also addresses the senses specifically:

> 厭目而視者視一以為兩
> 掩耳而聽者
> 聽漠漠而以為啕啕
> A person who presses the eye and looks, looks at one,[65] deeming it as two. A person who covers the ear and listens, listens to *mo-mo* but deems it as *hong-hong*.[66]
> (*Xunzi* 21/70)

In this explicit reference to sensory error, interference in the form of pressure from the hands diverts the senses from knowing.

Nothing in the *Xunzi* 21/70 passage implies that the senses' operations are inherently dubious. The passage *does* indicate a disparity between how things ordinarily look and how they can sometimes look; however, this disparity is not the difference between "things as they are" and "things as they seem to our senses." The cause of the error is a diversion in the direction of the normal effort to look and listen. The context of the rest of the passage—where darkness, distance, and alcohol affect things—also shows a disparity between things as they seem to the ordinary attention of the senses and things as they seem when sensory attention is misdirected. However, the passage presents the misdirected state as a rare occurrence, rather than as the normal state of affairs. It assumes that ordinarily, when we are not pressing on our eyes, we need raise no doubts about how we look at 'one.' Moreover, the passage blames the cause for doubt on unstable standards—or the undue influence of other things. The senses are not unreliable. The fault lies in the influence of things like an unstable heartmind, darkness, or blindness. The passage ends with the assertion that we should be careful about what we take as our standards. In terms of the senses, this frame implies that, like the heartmind (when it is stable), the senses are acceptable standards, provided other things do not interfere with them.

In *Xunzi* 21/70, sensory errors occur within the very act of listening and looking. These are not errors in hearing and seeing.[67] Although it does not translate well into English, the passage repeats the characters for "look" and "listen," rather than switching to "see" and "hear" in the second half of each line. It says that a person who puts pressure on his/her eye "looks at one, deeming it as two," instead of saying s/he "*looks* at one, but *sees* two." To understand the significance of this, we must investigate how listening and looking are distinguished from hearing and seeing in these texts.

In part, hearing and seeing refer to the completion of the effort represented by listening and looking.[68] Looking implies making an effort to pay attention, as in the following examples:

> 瞽者仰視而不見星
> Blind persons raise their heads and look, but do not see stars.
> (*Xunzi* 21/72–73)

The same is true of listening, which also indicates an exertion of effort:

> 各謹其所聞不務聽其所不聞
> 各謹其所見不務視其所不見
> Each is careful about what he hears, and does not *strive to listen* to what he does not hear. Each is careful about what he sees and does not *strive to look* at what he does not see.
> (*Xunzi* 11/111–112, emphasis added)

The notion that seeing and hearing indicate completion of this effort is evident in a variety of places. Just as "completion" is the terminus of "doing," the *Xunzi* says, ordinarily, seeing is the terminus of looking and hearing is the terminus of listening. The *Xunzi* condemns those who strain at looking and listening beyond their natural outcome:

> 是所謂視乎不可見
> 聽乎不可聞
> 為乎不可成
> This is what is called looking for what cannot be seen, listening for what cannot be heard, and *doing* what cannot be *completed.*
> (*Xunzi* 12/116–117, emphasis added)

By the same token, the *Xunzi*'s praise for exceptional people who can see without bothering to look also implies that seeing follows from the effort of looking:

> 不視而見
> [Such a person] does not look yet sees.
> (*Xunzi* 12/64, 24/2)

The *Mozi* also makes it clear that a certain amount of looking and listening constitutes an effort that normally produces a corresponding amount of seeing and hearing:

> 豈能一視而通見千里之外哉
> 一聽而通聞千里之外哉
> How were they [the sage-kings] able to see across a thousand *li* with one look? How were they able to hear across a thousand *li* with one [attempt at] listening?
> (*Mozi* 13/54)

Thus, part of the difference indicated by listening/looking versus hearing/seeing is the difference between making an effort and achieving a goal.

Aside from indicating effort, we might call the other feature of listening and looking "organizational." To look and listen is to organize things, in the sense of taking a certain attitude toward them. This is particularly obvious in certain uses of the terms. That is, *shi* 視 (look) can function as "to consider something to be something," and *ting* 聽 (listen) can function as "to judge." This explains why the person in *Xunzi* 21/70 can form a mistaken impression merely on the basis of looking and listening. Because *shi* functions as visually "consider" and *ting* functions as aurally "judge," looking and listening involve deeming things in certain ways.

Thus, sensory error can occur during the very effort to sense, which is an act of organizing the sensing in some particular direction. The fact that the error occurs during a process that is simultaneously the attempt to sense and a kind of deeming (effort and organization) rules out the perceptual model of error. That is, the error is not a matter of misreading the raw data caused by "things in themselves." It is not a miscalculated inference emerging at the completion of hearing and seeing. Because organizing already occurs during the effort to sense, there is no possibility of things giving rise to raw data that could be subject to interpretation. To use the examples from *Xunzi* 21/70, this depiction of sense discrimination does not present some "one" thing, sending out data, which is then misinterpreted as "two." Instead, it depicts the normal trajectory of looking—organizing in a visual effort—being misdirected by pressure on the eyes. So too, it does not present *mo-mo* data being misinterpreted as *hong-hong*. Instead, it depicts the normal trajectory of listening being deflected by pressure on the ears. The interference in the look's direction (which, in theory, could come from anything) changes the direction of the effort of sensing. The mistake is not due to misinterpretation—it is due to an obstruction of direction.

This treatment of sensory error in *Xunzi* 21/70 also makes sense discrimination seem like aspect perception. The notion that looking and listening are aimed at organizing things in a particular way resembles the continuous "seeing as" and "hearing as" of aspect perception. The organization is part of the senses' aim in one direction rather than another. In the very act of trying to look, the eyes look at something *as* something. As with aspect perception, the emphasis is on things *being regarded*. Indeed, the section of the passage begins with a person looking at "one" and listening to *mo-mo*.

The resemblance to aspect perception is also evident in the *Zhengming*'s description of the senses differentiating. This description occurs in the cause for difference section, which follows the cause for sameness. The cause for difference presents a much more detailed analysis of each sense operation:

> 形體色理以目異
> 聲音清濁調竽奇聲以耳異
> 甘苦鹹淡辛酸奇味以口異
> 香臭芬鬱腥臊洒酸奇臭以鼻異
> 疾養滄熱滑鈹輕重以形體異
> 説故喜怒哀樂愛惡欲以心異
>
> Forms, bodies, colors, and patterns are differentiated by the eye. Sounds and tones, clear and muddy, modes and harmony,[69] and strange sounds are differentiated by the ear. Sweet, bitter, salty, bland, pungent, sour, and strange tastes are differentiated by the mouth. Fragrances and stenches, perfumes and rotten odors, putrid and rancid

> smells, dank and sour smells,[70] as well as strange smells are differentiated by the nose. Illness and wellness,[71] cold and hot, smooth and sharp, light and heavy are differentiated by the form and body. Speech and causes,[72] happiness and anger, sadness and joy, loves, hates, and desires are differentiated by the heartmind.[73]
> (*Xunzi* 22/17–19)

These lists of things that are differentiated seem to cover the broadest possible range for each sense. The addition of "strange" sounds, tastes, and smells virtually guarantees that nothing is left out. Hence, the categories to be differentiated seem to designate each sense's range of possible forms of distinction.

This notion of differentiation implies something like aspect perception.[74] The categories that the senses differentiate are already too specific to suggest the sense data experienced by sensation. For example, tastes that are qualified enough to be called salty cannot be said to be raw sense data. At the same time, the reference to colors and shapes does not imply a perception model, wherein the senses take in data and the mind interprets it. The heartmind's role here is no different from the other senses. Each sense seems to perform its own differentiation within a system of contrasts.[75] In some cases, the contrasts are explicit. For example, the nose distinguishes between appealing fragrances and repulsive odors. Even when it is a question of differentiation among things that do not appear to have an opposite, like shapes, they are still determined by contrasts, because contrasts are inherent in the very notion of differentiating. Nothing can be differentiated without other things being rejected. Each selected differentiation inclines toward one direction and away from another (or others). Thus, the focus of attention in the passage is on a spectrum of humanly significant differentiations.

In saying that the *Xunzi* describes aspects of sense, I am not attributing a terribly complex view to the text. In spite of the fact that my explanation derives from Wittgenstein, it is not an extraordinary perspective. As Martin Heidegger points out, the complicated and abstract achievement is hearing sounds as distinct from whatever creates them:

> What we "first" hear is never noises or complexes of sounds, but the creaking waggon, the motorcycle. We hear the column on the march, the north wind, the woodpecker tapping, the fire crackling. It requires a very artificial and complicated frame of mind to "hear" a "pure noise."[76]

The discussion of sensory error in *Xunzi* 21/70 gives no indication that the *Xunzi* adopts such a complicated frame of mind that is required to think of sound as this kind of abstraction. The use of differentiate here reinforces that impression—the senses themselves are embedded in a context, and they discriminate among a spectrum of meaningful contrasts.

The fact that desirable conditions are often what the senses know corroborates this idea that the senses' knowledge is knowledge that is humanly significant. The senses know (or miss the opportunity to know) pleasure. For instance, in *Xunzi* 22/80 (see page 37), the mouth encounters the delicious taste of fine meat, but then fails to know it.[77] Similarly, in *Mozi* 32/6 (see page 37), the mouth encounters sweetness, and in this case *does* manage to know it. This knowing is directed in the sense of being attracted to a desire (and, consequently, away from an aversion). This is particularly evident in the examples of body knowledge from *Mozi* 32/5–6 and *Xunzi* 22/80–81. The body knows or fails to know what pleases it. In these examples, the body's knowledge is not something like the evidence of touch (determining whether something is or is not the case). Instead, the body knows the ease and comfort of desirable things, like temperate climates and bamboo mats. The knowledge implied in the metaphor of touch in the *Lunyu* 16/11 (where someone quickly removes his hand after touching boiling water) also seems to be a mastery of the reactions of attraction and repulsion. The touch of a hand rarely appears in lists of the senses, but when it does the context concerns desire.[78] In one of these rare cases referring to touch, the touch of the hands functions to signal the immensity of desired objects:

> 目不能遍視手不能遍操口不能遍味
> The eyes cannot see all the dishes, the hands cannot handle them all, and the mouth cannot taste them all.
> (*Mozi* 6/24–25)

The knowledge of the body, like the knowledge of the mouth, consists in knowing about the attraction of desirable things. Thus, sensory knowledge concerns attractions (and by implication, repulsions) appropriate to each sense. This is perhaps what the *Zhengming* means when it says that the senses have similar "intentional-things" (*yiwu* 意物) in response to similar things. In other words, it is not that they mechanically represent similar mental pictures of similar defining characteristics. Rather, they tend toward similarly attractive things and away from similarly repulsive things. Their discriminations manifest the context of human significance of which they are a part.

Verifying Knowledge

Verifying knowledge (the *Zhengming*'s term) is different from the knowledge I am calling sensory knowledge. Sensory knowledge applies to all of the senses (including the heartmind, because it too differentiates). Verifying knowledge is a feature of the heartmind involving the ears and the eyes for the purpose of verification.

The description of the causes for sameness and difference concludes with a brief comment on knowledge. Having just described the heartmind's differentiations, the passage adds,

> 心有徵知徵知則
> 緣耳而知聲可也
> 緣目而知形可也

> 然而徵知必將待天官當簿其類然後可也
> 五官簿之而不知心徵之而無説
> 則人莫不然謂之不知此所緣而以同異也
>
> The heartmind has verifying knowledge.[79] There is verifying knowledge; thus, because of [lit. caused by] the ear, it is possible to know sounds; because of [caused by] the eye, it is possible to know forms.[80] However, verifying must await the heavenly officials' meeting and recording their kinds in order to be possible. If the five officials record them without knowing, or if the heartmind verifies without speaking, then people will not fail to pronounce it "not knowing." It is this that causes sameness and difference.
> (*Xunzi* 22/19–21)

Much about this section is unclear. The subject seems to shift from the causes for sameness and difference to an explanation of the heartmind's verifying knowledge. The term "verifying knowledge" is unusual. It seems to involve only the heartmind, the eyes, and the ears.[81] The *Xunzi* adds a few more criteria necessary for knowledge to be recognized. Then, in spite of the focus on verifying knowledge, the last line reasserts that this is all part of the description of the causes of sameness and difference.[82]

As with the causes for sameness and difference, the model for this presentation of sensory knowledge is neither sensation nor perception. The participation of the heartmind rules out any resemblance to sensation. But the fact that the heartmind performs a verifying procedure involving the senses may initially sound like perception.[83] However, if I am correct in arguing above that form and sound are more like aspects than sense data, then the heartmind need not translate form and sound into something intelligible—as form aspects and sound aspects, they are already imbued with human significance.[84] The passage's attention to eliciting external confirmation of knowledge also differentiates it from a description of perception.[85] This emphasis on the heartmind's speaking implies a context of convincing others of one's knowledge, rather than a context of trying to arrive at certainty about what appears to the senses. The concern with getting others to concede that one knows brings a pragmatic element into the passage. Thus, insofar as this seems to be about verifying aspects rather than data, and insofar as it insists on corroboration from others, this picture of sense knowledge does not resemble sensation or perception.

Conclusions

Perhaps the ambiguities in this introductory overview reveal why sense discrimination in Warring States philosophical texts has never been the subject of lengthy sustained analysis: There are quite a few areas of indeterminacy in this portrait of sense discrimination. It is not certain whether there are only five senses, or which things count as senses. It is also not certain whether the senses are like well-structured government officials or a confused blend of openings, exposed to the vicissitudes of the wind.

Nevertheless, this study advances the theory that there are two different kinds of knowledge associated with the senses. In general, the senses know their discriminations, which are always embedded in a context of meaning. In addition, the heartmind, ears and eyes also participate in verifying knowledge.

Without eliminating the confusion, this overview does at least indicate where the confusion lies. Hopefully, it also points the reader in the right direction, with hypotheses that are grounded in the information, albeit fragmented, that is available.

Chapter 2: Hearing and Seeing

Of all the senses, hearing and sight appear most often in these texts. Like the senses as a whole, these two senses tend to appear in contexts related to knowledge or to desire. Because they appear in these similar contexts, the auditory and visual senses almost seem like substitutes for the senses as a whole. But the situation is more complex than this. Hearing and seeing play a unique role in the acquisition of knowledge. In my hypothesis, all of the senses may be described as knowing (insofar as they know what they desire), but hearing and seeing are significant for a particular form of knowing, that is, knowledge that pairs and tallies things. Moreover, as a result of this special role of hearing and seeing, aural and visual categories serve to divide the things in the world. A variety of things appear in aural and visual pairs within these texts. The variety and the relentlessness of these pairings imply that this bifurcation is fundamental to the way in which the universe is conceived. This should not be surprising: if knowledge (and sometimes desire) generally amounts to what is heard and seen, then the knower would inevitably tend to divide things into aural and visual categories. In other words, from the position that hearing and seeing constitute this important type of knowledge, the world itself should be something that is amenable to aural and visual bifurcation. And indeed, that is how the things in the world seem to appear in these texts.

Special Role of Hearing and Seeing

References to the desires of hearing and seeing do appear to serve as a synecdoche for all sensory desires. The *Xunzi* seems to use the ears and eyes to indicate the desires of the senses. For instance, it notes that the desires of the ears and eyes are present from birth:[1]

> 生而有耳目之欲
> 有好聲色焉
> 順之故淫亂生
> From birth, there are the desires of the ears and eyes—the fondness for sound and visual appearance [*se*][2]—the compliance with which causes the birth of looseness and chaos.
> (*Xunzi* 23/2)

Here, the desires of the ears and eyes probably represent all sensory desires, because it seems unlikely that other sensory desires are not also seen as present from birth. Similarly, the *Mozi* emphasizes the ears and eyes, when it describes the desires indulged in by wicked kings and avoided by the great sage king Yu.[3] Regarding the wicked kings, it says,

> 昔上世暴王不忍其耳目之淫心涂之辟
> In ages past, the wicked kings did not restrain the flowing of their ears and eyes and the deviance of their heartmind's pursuits.[4]
> (*Mozi* 35/38)

By contrast, according to the *Mozi,* satisfying the desires of the ears and eyes played no part at all in motivating the sage king Yu:

> 非以求以重富貴干福祿樂耳目也
> [King Yu did not go to war] on a quest to increase his wealth and status, to seek favor and fortune, or to please his ears and eyes.
> (*Mozi* 16/54–55)

The *Xunzi* also focuses on the ears and eyes, when noting the danger of rulers who aim to satisfy their desires:

> 其於聲色臺榭園囿也
> 愈厭而好新是傷國
> [If the ruler]—with regard to pleasant tones and good looks [*se*], pavilions and archery courts, parks, and gardens—requires more to be satisfied and is fond of newness, this harms the state.
> (*Xunzi* 11/132–133)

Like the *Mozi* and the *Xunzi*, the *Mencius* condemns indulging the desires of the ears and eyes, although it does so in the context of describing the social customs of ordinary people, rather than sage kings. According to the *Mencius*, following the desires of the ears and eyes is one among five things that society considers unfilial (see *Mencius* 4B30 in Chapter 1, footnote 22). In each of these cases, there seems to be no particular reason for the emphasis on the desires of the ears and eyes, rather than, say, the mouth. Thus, the passage suggests that, insofar as the senses of hearing and seeing seek pleasures and must be restrained, they may represent all sensory desires.

Like these contexts describing desire, the senses of the ears and eyes are highlighted in contexts related to knowledge. In many cases, they represent knowledge itself. The phrase "to hear and see" actually can be interpreted as "to know" or "to understand." For instance, noble people are those who hear and see (understand) beyond the scope of their listening and looking:

> 君子...心小而道大
> 所聽視者近而所聞見者遠
> As for noble people...their heartminds are small but their way is great; what they listen for and look at is near, but what they hear and see is far.[5]
> (*Xunzi* 3/35)

The ability to hear and see is an achievement that forms the completion of listening and looking and transforms them into knowing. In fact, at every level of the achievement of knowledge, these texts invoke hearing and seeing. In brief, the picture of knowledge looks like this: those who know nothing can neither hear nor see (*Mozi* 46/3–4 and *Zhuangzi* 1/30–31); the knowledge of a cultivated scholar is limited to hearing and seeing (*Xunzi* 8/96); the understanding of spiritual beings is marked by heightened hearing and seeing (*Mozi* 46/3–4);[6] and the greatest knowledge need not rely on what is already heard and seen (*Xunzi* 8/98–99 and *Lunyu* 7/28).

Starting at the bottom of this hierarchy, according to the *Mozi*, the deaf and the blind are the least knowledgeable of all:

> 鬼神之明智於聖人猶聰耳明目之與聾瞽也
> The clear understanding of ghosts and spirits, in relation to that of the sages, is like the sharp eared and keen sighted with regard to the deaf and blind.
> (*Mozi* 46/3–4)

The *Zhuangzi* expresses a similar assumption that the inability to understand is a kind of deafness or blindness. In a dialogue where one character fails to appreciate something, the other character casts his failure in terms of blindness and deafness. He says,

> 然瞽者無以與乎文章之觀
> 聾者無以與乎鐘鼓之聲
> 豈唯形骸有聾盲哉夫知亦有之
> Yes, the blind lack what is needed to share in the spectacle of emblems and ornaments, and the deaf lack what is needed to share in the sound of drums and bells. Is it only form and bone that has blindness and deafness? The knowledge also has them.
> (*Zhuangzi* 1/30–31)

By itself, this comparison of knowledge's failure to blindness and deafness implies that knowledge amounts to appreciating beauty and music. However, in combination, the two references to deafness and blindness make a less specific point: that knowledge depends on being able to see and hear.

Moreover, the *Xunzi* and the *Lunyu* also measure knowledge through the senses of hearing and seeing, by drawing a distinction between what they consider the highest two levels of knowledge. To highlight the difference between the "elegant" scholars and those who are even greater, the *Xunzi* contrasts two types of knowledge in terms of their capacities for hearing and seeing. Although it ranks the elegant scholars over the common people and the vulgar scholars, it notes that the knowledge of elegant scholars is restricted to patterns that are based on what they have already heard and seen:

> 聞見之所未至
> 則知不能類也
> What their hearing and seeing has not reached, their knowledge cannot classify.
> (*Xunzi* 8/96)

This amounts to no great insult, because the *Xunzi does* credit these elegant scholars with knowledge. However, the knowledge of truly great scholars is more independent:

> 所未嘗聞也
> 所未嘗見也
> 卒然起一方
> 則舉統類而應之
> Regarding that which they have not heard and that which they have not seen—if one corner is suddenly held up, they can pick out the whole classification and respond to it.[7]
> (*Xunzi* 8/98–99)

In other words, what these great scholars have heard or seen constitutes the sum of what they already know, but they need not depend on such past knowledge. The *Lunyu* makes a similar point about knowledge that is not bound to the past. The passage presents Confucius as saying that the ultimate form of knowing is initiating something without knowing it:

> 蓋有不知而作之者我無是也
> 多聞擇其善者而從之多見而識之
> 知之次也
> There may be those who, unknowingly, create things. I am not like this. Those who hear much, select the good, and follow it; those who see much, and remember it—this is the next kind of knowing.
> (*Lunyu* 7/28)

This passage identifies hearing and sight with knowing, while conceding the possibility of another kind of knowing. Not deeming himself capable of the highest kind of knowing, Confucius seems to place himself among those who hear and see much. These distinctions between the two most advanced levels of knowledge reiterate the importance of hearing and seeing for knowing: while some may know what they have not yet heard or seen, ordinarily, knowledge is what has already been heard and seen.

Furthermore, the use and rejection of these two senses—in the *Mozi* and the *Zhuangzi*, respectively—represent the use and rejection of knowledge itself. For instance, the *Mozi* invokes the ears and eyes of the common people as one of the three factors that contribute to establishing standards for knowledge. (Utility and the concerns of the sages are the two other contributing factors.) Proposing the means for establishing standards, the *Mozi* asks,

> 於何本之上本之於古者聖王之事
> 於何原之下原察百姓耳目之實
> 於何用之廢以為刑政觀其中國家
> 百姓人民之利

> How are they to be based? They should be based on the concerns of the ancient sage kings. How are they to be originated? They are to be originated by products of the ears and eyes of the common people.[8] How are they to be applied? They are to be applied by adopting them in government and observing their benefits to the country and the hundred surnames.
> (*Mozi* 35/8–9)

Various forms of this appeal to the ears and eyes appear repeatedly in the text of the *Mozi*.[9] According to the *Mozi*, the method of knowing whether or not something exists is to use the product of the masses' ears and eyes as one's instrument of measure:

> 是與天下之所以察知有與無之道者
> 必以眾之耳目之實知有與亡為儀者也
> 請惑聞之見之則必以為有
> 莫聞莫見則必以為無
> Now as to the way to check to know whether or not a thing exists, it is to take as one's instrument the product of the ears and eyes of the multitude. If, indeed, some have heard it or seen it, then we have to say it is there. If no one has heard it and no one has seen it, then we have to say it not there.
> (*Mozi* 31/10–11)

The *Mozi* considers objections to its emphasis on the ears and eyes of the masses, but even the objections do not question the importance of hearing and seeing for knowing. Instead, they pose doubts about whether the masses themselves ought to be trusted. Granting that the masses could be unreliable, the *Mozi* addresses this objection by considering what the feudal lords have heard and seen:

> 若以百姓為愚不肖耳目之情不足因而為法
> 然則胡不嘗考之諸侯之傳言流語乎

> 自古以及今生民以來者
> 亦嘗有聞命之聲見命之體者乎
> 則未嘗有也
> If the common people are considered stupid and worthless, and the *qing* [conditions? dispositions?] of their ears and eyes are not reliable as a standard, then why not inquire into the recorded speech of the feudal lords that has flowed down to us? From olden times until now, from the time that people have been born, has any of them *heard* the sound of *ming* [fate/ordainment/decree] or *seen* the body [*ti*] of *ming*? Of course, none of them has.
> (*Mozi* 36/7–9, emphasis added)

Thus, even if relying on the hearing and seeing of the masses seems dubious, one can rely on the hearing and seeing of the feudal lords. This attention to the feudal lords' hearing and seeing confirms the importance of these two senses for the *Mozi*'s view of knowledge. Moreover, the fact that the feudal lords' hearing and seeing trumps that of the masses sheds light on what the appeal to the "ears and eyes of the masses" really means. The fact that the *Mozi* is quite willing to abandon the ears and eyes of the masses in favor of those of the nobles suggests that the source of knowledge in the repeated phrase "ears and eyes of the masses" is not certitude about listening and looking. The masses may be wrong about what they hear and see. The argument ultimately only trusts the hearing and seeing of those to whom tradition attributes knowledge, and it seems to do so primarily in the interests of utility—as if this is what it takes to convince its audience. Thus, these two senses operate as standards for establishing knowledge only in combination with the other two criteria—utility and the wisdom of the ancient sages.

Perhaps deliberately echoing the *Mozi*'s refrain of "the ears and eyes of the masses," the *Zhuangzi* seems to dismiss knowledge, specifically by rejecting the eyes and ears of the masses. In the

Zhuangzi's unconventional perspective, the sages disregard the masses' ears and eyes, as well as their own eyes and ears:

> 忘其肝膽遺其耳目反覆終始不知端倪
> 芒然彷徨乎塵垢之外逍遙乎無為之業
> 彼又惡能憒憒然為世俗之禮
> 以觀眾人之耳目哉
> [These sages…] forget their liver and gall, abandon their ears and eyes. They turn and repeat, end and begin, without knowing their starting point or origin. They forgetfully ramble outside the dust and dirt, wandering through the instructions of non-action.
> How could they even be capable of fussily performing the rituals of the world for the ears and eyes of the multitude?
> (*Zhuangzi* 6/69–71)

After abandoning these senses, these sages seem genuinely confused. The passage above stresses that they do not know the most basic of distinctions. In fact, each mention of abandoning hearing and seeing in the *Zhuangzi* is followed by some form of rejection of knowledge. For example, in the parodic dialogue between a fictionalized Confucius and his pupil Yan Hui, the loss of knowledge appears immediately after loss of perspicacity in seeing and hearing. Yan Hui summarizes his (meditative?) practice of "sitting and forgetting" in these terms:

> 墮肢體黜聰明離形去知
> 同於大通此謂坐忘
> I drop off limbs and trunk, dismiss keenness of hearing and clarity of eyesight, leave form and expel knowledge, and unite with the great thoroughfare. This is what I mean by "sitting and forgetting."
> (*Zhuangzi* 6/92–93)

Likewise, the *Zhuangzi* praises sages for not knowing what is appropriate to ears and eyes, which then causes their heartminds (the function in charge of a certain kind of knowing) to roam:

> 夫若然者且不知耳目之所宜
> 而遊心乎德之和
> As for such people, they do not know what is appropriate to the ears and eyes, and they cause their heartminds to roam in the peace of *de* [charisma/virtue].
> (*Zhuangzi* 5/7–8)

Indeed, permitting the heartmind to roam does seem to mean expelling its knowledge. In another fictionalized dialogue between Confucius and Yan Hui, Confucius hints that following the channels of the ears and eyes leads straight to the loss of the heartmind's knowledge:

> 夫徇耳目內通
> 而外於心知
> 鬼神將來舍而況人乎
> 是萬物之化也
> If you accord with the inward circulation through the eyes and ears, and externalize the heartmind's knowing, the *gui* [ghostly] and *shen* [spiritual] will come and reside, and all the more so the human![10]
> (*Zhuangzi* 4/32–33)

When read in light of the other ear and eye references, the "according" with the inward channels of the ears and eyes in this passage suggests some kind of refusal to hear and see.[11] Once again, this is succeeded by dismissing the heartmind—specifically its knowledge. Thus, once again, a reference to ears and eyes indicates knowledge. In sum, in sharp contrast to the *Mozi*, the *Zhuangzi* rejects the eyes and ears and thereby rejects the knowledge they represent.[12]

Perhaps as a result of their role in acquiring knowledge, hearing and seeing also represent the height of human powers throughout these texts. An acute capacity for hearing and seeing seems to coincide with a condition of physical strength. The individuals who have the sharpest capacities of hearing and sight are in their physical prime, according to the *Mozi*. In its criticism of the misuse of music, the *Mozi* notes that rulers require people in their prime to play it, because the very young and the very old have inferior capacities of hearing and sight.[13] Apparently, the weak limbs of youth and old age are accompanied by diminished capacities of hearing and sight. In addition to youth and old age, the *Mozi* also notes that powers of hearing and sight are damaged by the process of mourning (a phenomenon also described in the *Mencius*). The fact that mourning damages the ability to hear and see seems to be a tribute to the extremity of the sacrifice that mourning calls forth. The *Mencius* discusses the case of a certain person who fasts for three days, and thereupon loses his hearing and sight:

> …三日不食耳無聞目無見
> …after three days of not eating, his ears lacked the ability to hear, his eyes lacked the ability to see.
> (*Mencius* 3B10)

While the *Mencius* proffers qualified praise for such behavior (it does note that the admirable severity of such mourning cannot guarantee integrity), the *Mozi* explicitly criticizes it. In the *Mozi*'s critique (which turns three days into three years), losing these powers of hearing and sight renders the mourner worthless:

> 三年哭泣
> 扶後起杖後行
> 耳無聞目無見

> Crying and weeping lasts for three years. They need a cane to stand up and a cane to walk. Their ears lack [the ability to] hear and their eyes lack [the ability to] see.
> (*Mozi* 48/51)

Whether cited with approval or condemnation, the fact that damage to the ears and eyes serves as the measure of the extremity of one's sacrifice implies that the capacities of hearing and sight are of supreme value. Moreover, like the reference to hearing and eyesight being weakened during old age and youth, these descriptions of the effects of mourning make the point that these senses function best when the body as a whole is strong. Thus, conditions that undermine the vitality of the entire body likewise undermine the capacities of hearing and seeing. In sum, well-functioning senses of hearing and sight coincide with maximally healthy and vital human powers.

This connection of hearing and sight with power may explain why the capacities of these two senses are necessary for unifying the empire. In the *Mozi*'s mythic reconstruction of the past, a wise emperor makes a statement implying that only his ears and eyes prevent him from being able to unify the world by himself:

> 天子既以立矣
> 以為唯其耳目之請
> 不能獨一同天下之義
> 是故選擇天下贊閱賢良聖知辯慧之人
> Upon becoming established, the emperor—taking the *qing* [conditions? dispositions?] of his own ears and eyes as incapable of unifying the world—selected the world's experienced, virtuous, intelligent, and wise people [and installed them].
> (*Mozi* 12/7)

Similarly, the *Mencius* also contains a myth describing ancient sages who require supplementary powers of hearing and sight in order to benefit the world:

> 聖人既竭目力焉
> 繼之以規矩準繩以為方員平直不可勝用
> 既竭耳力焉
> 繼之以六律正五音不可勝用焉
> 既竭心思焉
> 繼之以不忍人之政而仁覆天下矣
> When the sages had exhausted the strength of their eyes, they followed that with the compass, the square, the level, and the line, which could be inexhaustibly used to make things square, round, level, and straight.
> When they had exhausted the strength of their ears, they followed that with the pitch tubes, which could be inexhaustibly used to set in order the five notes.
> When they had exhausted their heartmind's thinking, they followed that with a government that could not endure human suffering—and benevolence overspread the kingdom.
> (*Mencius* 4A1)

In both these passages, the inadequacy of hearing and seeing seems to indicate that an *individual's* powers are insufficient to the task. The scope of any one individual's hearing and sight is too limited, as the *Mozi* points out:

> 是故古之聖王之治天下也
> 千里之外有賢人焉其鄉里之人皆未之均聞見也
> 聖王得而賞之....
> 故唯毌以聖王為聰耳明目與
> 豈能一視而通見千里之外哉
> 一聽而通聞千里之外哉
> 聖人不往而視之 不就而聽之

> Therefore, in the ancient sage kings' ordering of the world, if there were good people more than a thousand *li* away,[14] they would be able to reward them before all those who were within their own villages heard and saw [their goodness].... Only do not take the sage kings as having done so with their own keen ears and clear eyes. How could they be able to see across a thousand *li* with one look? How could they be able to hear across a thousand *li* with one [attempt at] listening? The sages look at things without going, listen to things without approaching them.
> (*Mozi* 13/51–55)

As both the *Mencius* and *Mozi* passages suggest, a single individual's hearing and sight is limited in range. Moreover, from the *Xunzi* we find that hearing and sight are also limited in their ability to focus (that is, *Xunzi* 1/22 says it is impossible to focus the ears and eyes on more than one thing at once).[15] Thus, the advantage of things like compasses, pitch tubes, and the assistance of multiple ears and eyes is that they expand the scope of an individual's knowledge. The ability to hear and see an area means having knowledge of it and the power to control it. Hence, hearing and seeing are essential to unifying the empire, because they represent the ability to know—and thereby the power to control— that which falls within their range.

The Heard and the Seen

In addition to their unique connection to knowledge, hearing and seeing are distinct from the other senses in their effect on how the world is construed. Along with the prominence of seeing and hearing comes a prominence of things heard and seen. Even if one holds the view that hearing and seeing merely serve as a synecdoche for the senses as a whole, the effects are striking. The sensed world is generally met by hearing and seeing, instead of being contacted by a variety of senses. In effect, the world seems to present itself in terms of this bifurcation—as things to be either heard or seen.

For instance, the objects of desire tend to be either aural or visual. These items are not fixed—the ears and eyes are described as desiring different things in different contexts. The variety of items that match the ears' and eyes' desires suggests that the pattern of aurality and visuality is more significant than the items involved. *Xunzi* 11/132 (see page 52) remarks that the ears and eyes desire pleasant tones and good looks. The *Lunyu* phrases this slightly differently: it quotes Confucius as criticizing his generation for its emphasis on eloquence and beauty:

> 子曰不有祝鮀之佞而有宋朝之美
> 難乎免於今之世矣
> Without the eloquence of Priest Tuo or the beauty of Song Chao, it is difficult to avoid danger in this present age.
> (*Lunyu* 6/16)

The objects of desire cited in the *Mencius* 1B1 present another variation on the aural and visual, reflecting the context of a royal hunt. The ruler's desire for hunting is observed by the people, who overhear the pounding of the ruler's horses' hooves and catch sight of the beauty of the hunt's ornamentation. Mencius says to a king,

> 今王田獵於此百姓聞王車馬之音
> 見羽旄之美...而相告曰吾王之好田獵
> Now when your Majesty hunts like this, the common people hear the noise of your carriages and horses and see the beauty of your plumes and streamers...and speak to each other of "our king's love of hunting...."
> (*Mencius* 1B1)

Here in the context of enjoying a hunt, the ears wish to hear pounding hooves and the eyes wish to see the ornaments of the hunt. As this last example shows clearly, in different cases, the specified objects of the ears and eyes' desires can vary.[16] But these variations highlight the importance of the pattern—in each case, the world of desire consists of some form of aural and visual pairs.

The combination of the heard and the seen indicates something else when used to describe human beings. The aural and the visual constitute the impression of a person as a whole. For example, the *Mencius* sums up the dangers of arrogance in terms of a person's tone and look:

> 訑訑之聲音顏色距人於千里之外
> The tone and look of arrogance will keep people away as far as a thousand *li*.
> (*Mencius* 6B13)

> 恭儉豈可以聲音笑貌為哉
> Respectfulness and restraint: how can these be obtained from tone of voice and a smiling demeanor?
> (*Mencius* 4A17)

This distrust of tone and appearance seems to derive from the *Mencius*'s theory that the heartmind's concerns will manifest themselves in a similar aural/visual pair:

> 人恆過然後能改困於心衡於慮而後作徵於色發於聲而後喻
> Generally, people are able to learn after they make mistakes. Only after their heartminds feel surrounded and their thoughts feel crossed, are [people able] to create. Only after being evident in their looks and issued in their voices, are things clear.
> (*Mencius* 6B15)

Thus, it is fitting that in the *Mencius*, when spectators come to view the sincerity of someone's mourning, they attend to the sound of their cries and the look on their face:

> 四方來觀之
> 顏色之戚哭泣之哀弔者大悦
> They came from all quarters to observe it. The mourners were greatly pleased by the miserable look on his face and the pathos of his crying and weeping.
> (*Mencius* 3A2)

The *Mozi* uses similar categories to indicate familiarity with a person. *Mozi* is quoted as saying,

> 吾非與之並世同時親聞其聲見其色也
> I am no contemporary of theirs, neither have I heard their sounds nor seen their countenances.
> (*Mozi* 16/49)

While the *Lunyu* makes a similar kind of claim about human appearances, it specifically emphasizes a person's speech, rather than the more general terms for "sound." (The pairing of speech with something else—action—will be discussed in detail below.) Two quotations attributed to Confucius both use people's speech and looks to refer to their general appearance:

> 巧言令色鮮矣仁
> It is rare for clever speech and an insinuating look to accompany benevolence.
> (*Lunyu* 1/3)

> 察言而觀色
> [A person of achievement] examines people's speech and observes their countenances.
> (*Lunyu* 12/20)

The pattern is so pervasive that the same pair of terms even applies to meeting an animal in the *Mencius*. The *Mencius* explains that if noble people hear or see an animal, they will feel too familiar with it to permit it to die:

> 君子之於禽獸也見其生不忍見其死聞其聲不忍食其肉
> Such is the noble person's attitude towards animals: having seen them alive, they cannot bear to see them die; having heard their cries, they cannot bear to eat their flesh. (*Mencius* 1A7)

The heard and the seen represent everything significant in appearance. Just as the desired objects of the eyes and ears take a variety of forms, so too the aural and visual aspects of animals and humans differ. But this difference merely reinforces the point—the aural and visual pairs themselves matter more than the content of those pairs.

Speech and Action

In addition to providing a way to sum up human appearances, hearing and seeing also provide knowledge of human character. The emphasis on these two senses is not arbitrary, because hearing and seeing sense the two things whose correspondence is the foundation for knowledge about humans, that is, the ears hear speech, and the eyes see action. And when speech matches action, like two parts of a tally, it becomes possible to trust and know.

As the examples from the *Lunyu* show (1/3, 12/20), references to hearing are not confined to sensing sounds per se—references to hearing also indicate hearing speech and its content. In other words, the "object" of hearing includes speech, as well as the actual sound of the voice. In fact, the character "sound" itself sometimes refers to speech. For example, in different contexts in the *Mencius*, the same term (*sheng*) refers to both the physical sound of the voice and the speech it articulates. After Confucius dies, his disciples are said to "lose sound."

> 相嚮而哭皆失聲
> They turned towards one another and cried until they all lost their voices [*sheng*].
> (*Mencius* 3A4)

The same term for sound also functions as speech in the case where someone has a retort for any bad sounds directed at him:

> 惡聲至必反之
> Any bad word [*sheng*] that reached him, he always returned.
> (*Mencius* 2A2)

Sometimes, the sound of the voice seems to overlap with the speech it conveys. For instance, the *Mencius* does not really distinguish *sheng* from *yan* when it says of Bo Yi, in two different places, that he would not listen to a bad *sound* and that he would not *speak* to a bad person. Both instances remark that Bo Yi would not serve a bad ruler, and both mention that there is something sensed by hearing that Bo Yi would not do. Thus, the *Mencius* seems to be rephrasing, when it says the following two things:

> 伯夷目不視惡色耳不聽惡聲非其君不事
> Bo Yi's eyes would not look at bad [visual] appearances, and his ears would not listen to bad sounds. If it was not his prince, he would not serve him.
> (*Mencius* 5B1)

> 不立於惡人之朝
> 不與惡人言
> [of Bo Yi] He would not stand in a bad prince's court, and he would not speak with a bad person.
> (*Mencius* 2A9)

These examples from the *Mencius* confirm that hearing sounds sometimes functions as the equivalent of hearing speech in these texts.[17] Thus, it seems reasonable that the object of hearing may be sound or speech.

When the object of hearing is speech, the corresponding object of vision is usually action.[18] The idea that action is visible to the eyes is asserted in this passage from the *Xunzi*:[19]

> 言為可聞
> 行為可見
> Speech is what it is possible to hear.
> Action is what it is possible to see.
> (*Xunzi* 27/87–88)

It is also indicated by one case in the *Lunyu*, which likewise implies that observation of action is the visual counterpart to hearing speech. In describing how Confucius hopes to escape errors, it says,

> 今吾於人也
> 聽其言而觀其行
> Nowadays, in my dealings with others, upon listening to their speech, I observe their actions.
> (*Lunyu* 5/10)

This suggestion that action is visible becomes more explicit when read in conjunction with another section of the *Lunyu*. In a passage similarly concerned with avoiding errors, in the same way that listening normally precedes hearing, the *Lunyu* asserts that looking should precede acting:

> 多聞闕疑慎言其餘則寡尤
> 多見闕殆慎行其餘則寡悔
> If you listen broadly, set aside what you are unsure of, and speak cautiously on the rest, you will make few errors; if

> you look broadly, set aside what is perilous, and act cautiously on the rest, you will have few regrets.
> (*Lunyu* 2/18)

These lines suggest not only that speech and action are sensed by the ears and eyes, respectively, but that speech and action are primary objects associated with these two senses. In the context of observing human beings, while speech is the frequent corollary of hearing, its matching visual corollary is usually action.

The reason action is construed as being sensed by vision is that action literally refers to walking, which is more accessible to vision than to any other sense. The character *xing* 行 functions to mean both "walk" and, by extension, "act." Moreover, walking creates paths and leaves footsteps that are visible to the eyes. A reference to looking at someone treading a path appears in a passage from the *Shi Jing*, which is cited in both the *Mozi* and the *Mencius*. The petty person looks (at the walking or at the path being walked), whereas the noble person walks a path:

> 其直若矢其易若底
> 君子之所履小人之所視
> It [the ruler's way] is straight like an arrow and smooth like a whetstone. The noble person treads it; the petty person looks upon it.[20]
> (*Mozi* 16/61)

The *Mencius*'s use of the same passage expands the visual metaphor, by suggesting that the ruler, like the petty people, also watches a noble person who treads the way. This case from the *Mencius* discusses how a virtuous person should be summoned to go to court. It compares seeing virtuous people with wanting them to walk through a gate—if one wants to see them, one must provide the proper road and gate:

> 欲見賢人而不以其道猶欲其入而閉之門也
> 夫義路也禮門也惟君子能由是路出入是門也
> 詩云周道如底其直如矢君子所履小人所視
> When a ruler desires to *see* people of virtue, but does not use this [proper] way, it is like wanting them to enter [the palace] and shutting the gate against them. Now, righteousness is the road, and ritual is the gate, but only noble persons can follow this way, entering and exiting this gate. The *Book of Poetry* says, "The way to Zhou is like a whetstone, and straight as an arrow. The noble person treads it; the petty person looks upon it."
> (*Mencius* 5B7)

This Mencian extrapolation of the *Shi Jing* passage implies that action is visible, by alluding to the motion of walking through a gate as well as the traces created by treading a path. A passage from the *Mozi* even uses the metaphor of "following in footsteps" of someone's actions as the counterpart for hearing their speech.

> 聖人聽其言跡其行察其所能...
> The sages listened to their speech, retraced their actions, and examined their capabilities...
> (*Mozi* 9/6)

Hence, action amounts to walking, which creates motion and other traces that can be seen by the eyes. Thus, just as speech may be heard by the ears, the act of walking may be seen by the eyes.

Given these parallels between audible speech and visible action, it is not surprising that hearing and seeing play a special role in gaining knowledge of human character. Human beings can be known through their speech and action, especially if the two tally with one another. But, according to these texts, knowledge based on either speech or action alone is precarious, as I will explain below.[21] Only speech and action that tally suffice for knowing people.

The parallels between speech and action in these texts suggest that these two things constitute the most significant features of a human being. In its ranking of levels of scholar officials, the *Lunyu* implies that ordinary people value trustworthy speech and productive action. Confucius himself is not terribly impressed by these values; he calls them "stubborn" and ranks them third, following those who act without disgracing their rulers and those who act with filial piety. Yet he offers this telling description of "the little people":

> 言必信行必果硜硜然小人哉
> They are determined to be trustworthy in what they say and make sure their actions have results—stubborn little people.
> (*Lunyu* 13/20)

The *Mencius* extrapolates on the point, suggesting that "great" people have no such aim to be trustworthy in speech or productive in action.

> 大人者言不必信行不必果
> 惟義所在
> Great people's speech need not be trustworthy, and their actions need not be productive. They simply need to reside in righteousness.
> (*Mencius* 4B11)

But this comment from the *Mencius* does not deny that the little people do indeed need to be trustworthy in speech and productive in action. Nor does it deny that the great people actually are trustworthy in speech and productive in action. It only denies that among great people this requires any effort beyond being righteous. Thus, these passages from the *Lunyu* and the *Mencius* ultimately affirm the prevalence of the value of trustworthy speech and productive action in these texts.[22]

Aside from these passages from the *Lunyu* and the *Mencius*, repeated attention to speech and action elsewhere confirms the value placed on these two things. The *Zhuangzi* notes that speech and action put a person's character to the test. The *Zhuangzi* says,

> 言者風波也行者實喪也
> 夫風波易以動
> 實喪易以危
> Speech is wind and waves,
> Action is fulfillment and loss.
> It is easy for wind and waves to move [things], and as easy for fulfillment and loss to endanger [things].
> (*Zhuangzi* 4/49–50)

Thus, speech and action present a challenge: they are the means by which people are swayed and tempted to danger. Hence they are the focus of character building and the focus of assessing the character of others. The *Mozi* recommends assimilating the speech and action of virtuous people in order to become virtuous oneself.[23] Sagacity and virtue manifest themselves in speech and action. In its explanation for why Confucius was not a virtuous person, a character in the *Mozi* offers this conception of being virtuous:[24]

> 是以言明而易知也
> 行明而易從也
> It is this: their speech is clear and easy to understand.
> Their actions are clear and easy to follow.
> (*Mozi* 39/39)

The *Lunyu* and the *Mencius* do not disagree with this emphasis on the speech and action of the virtuous (although they would surely disagree that Confucius does not fit them). In fact, the *Lunyu* reports that Confucius explains proper action in these terms:

> 言忠信行篤敬雖蠻貊之邦行矣
> Your speech should be reliable and trustworthy, and your actions should be straightforward and respectful—[so you should] act, even in the foreign nations of the Man or Mo.
> (*Lunyu* 15/6)

The *Lunyu* focuses on the same qualifications to justify deeming two officials to be virtuous in spite of their having risked disgrace:

> 言中倫行中慮
> [of Hui of Liu Xia and Shao Lian] Their speech was on target with analysis and their actions were on target with pondering.
> (*Lunyu* 18/8)

The *Lunyu* also criticizes people by focusing on flaws in their speech and action:

> 群居終日言不及義好行小慧難矣哉
> If you get together a number of people and all day their speech never reaches [the subject of] righteousness, while they adore acting on petty shrewdness: that's a difficult case.
> (*Lunyu* 15/7)

The *Mencius* uses the same categories to establish the presence or absence of virtue in a variety of circumstances. The *Mencius* cites a conversation wherein one of Mencius's dialogue partners uses these categories to assess Confucius and his followers. The comment evaluates all of them in terms of their speech and/or action:[25]

> 宰我子貢善為説辭
> 冉牛閔子顏淵善言德行
> 孔子兼之曰吾於辭命則不能也

> Zaiwo and Zigong were good at speaking/explaining rhetoric, Ran Niu, Minzi, and Yan Hui, were good at speaking and virtuous in acting.[26] Confucius united these traits, yet he said, "With regard to rhetoric, I am not capable."
> (*Mencius* 2A2)

The same categories for evaluation also emerge from the mouth of Mencius himself, when he is cited as providing this description of the ancient sage, Shun:

> 聞一善言見一善行若決江河沛然
> 莫之能禦也
> When he heard a single good word, or saw a single good action, he was like the bursting of a stream or a river, so overwhelming that none could withstand it.
> (*Mencius* 7A16)

Mencius himself is also cited as noting the role of speech and action in determining whether noble persons should serve a ruler. Of old, noble persons would serve on the condition that the ruler promised to enact their speech:

> 言將行其言也則就之
> 禮貌未衰言弗行也則去之
> [If the ruler] said he was going to put their speech into practice, then they would go to him. If, without ritual or manners diminishing, their speech was not put into practice, then they would leave him.
> (*Mencius* 6B14)

Occasionally, a third element enters the equation, but the point is essentially the same. For instance, the *Mencius* tacks on clothes to a claim that otherwise says that speech and action make the person:

> 服堯之服誦堯之言行堯之行是堯而已矣
> Wear the clothes of Yao, recite the words of Yao, and do the actions of Yao, and you will just be a Yao.
> (*Mencius* 6B2)

Similarly, the *Mozi* supplies the factor of government, in addition to speech and action, to the list of criteria for determining the presence of righteousness:

> 觀其行順天之意謂之善意行反天之意謂之不善意行觀其言談順天之意謂之善言談反天之意謂之不善言談觀其刑政順天之意謂之善刑政反天之意謂之不善刑政
> Observe people's actions, and if they accord with the intent of heaven, call them well–intended actions. If they are contrary to the intent of heaven, call them not well–intended actions. Observe their speech and talk, if they accord with the intent of heaven, call them good speech and talk. If they are contrary to the intent of heaven, call them bad speech and talk. Observe their laws and government, if they accord with the intent of heaven, call them well–intended laws and government. If they are contrary to the intent of heaven, call them bad laws and government.
> (*Mozi* 27/69–71)

Even with the addition of things like clothes and government, the pattern of emphasis on speech and action is clear. For the purposes of character evaluation, the two significant features of a human being are speech and action. They provide the basis for determining whether or not a person is virtuous. Thus, they provide all that needs to be known about the character of others.

Yet speech and action are not automatically reliable sources of knowledge. The most common obstruction to correct evaluation of speech and action is a lack of equivalence between them—a condition particularly likely to result from an excess on the part of speech. The texts commonly indict speech for surpassing action.[27] Apparently, it is easier for speech to exceed action than vice versa. Speech can seem reckless and careless. The *Zhuangzi* contrasts it with the more dignified act of walking the way. For example, when commenting on a description of a sage, one follower of Confucius says,

> 夫子以為孟浪之言
> 而我以為妙道之行也
> The Master took this [description] to be speech of careless extravagance. I take it to be walking of the most excellent way.
> (*Zhuangzi* 2/75)

This recklessness may express itself in a tendency to bypass action. The *Lunyu* calls this a source of shame:

> 恥其言而過其行
> The gentleman is ashamed lest he speak and thereby overpass his action.
> (*Lunyu* 14/27)

As the *Mozi* puts it, a person consists of a mouth that speaks and a body that acts. By speaking, it is possible for the mouth to create chaos in the body:[28]

> 政者口言之身必行之
> 今子口言之而身不行
> 是子之身亂也
> 子不能治子之身惡能治國政
> In governing, what the mouth speaks, the body must enact. Now your mouth says something, but your body does not act [on it]. This is your body being in chaos. If you cannot

govern your body, how can you govern the administration of a state?
(*Mozi* 48/85–86)

Taken rather literally, speech seems to flow out from the mouth and travel to places where action cannot catch up to it:

古者言之不出恥躬之不逮也
The ancients did not emit speech, because they would be ashamed lest they would not personally be able to pursue what they said.
(*Lunyu* 4/22)

It is as if speech has a certain speed that, in some cases, needs to be counteracted by slowing speech down, while quickening the pace of action:[29]

君子欲訥於
言而敏於行
The exemplary person wants to be slow to speak, yet quick to act.
(*Lunyu* 4/24)

In sum, speech has a certain fluidity that action lacks. Perhaps this is because, in addition to covering a broader ranger of space, the texts suggest that sound also carries faster than its visual counterpart.[30] Action often seems obliged to pursue speech, in an attempt to create or restore order.

To counteract the speed of sound, there is a recurring tendency to measure speech and action against one another in these texts. If one allows a disparity between speech and action, the consequences are dire. People will cease paying attention:

務言而緩行
雖辯必不聽

> As for those who make every effort to speak but are slow to act, even if they are discerning, no one will listen.
> (*Mozi* 2/12)

Thus, the *Mozi* seeks only speech that can affect action. The rest, it says, is a waste of the mouth.[31] The *Xunzi* also objects to wasting the mouth, which is exemplified by an incongruity between saying and doing.[32] Furthermore, it criticizes those whose mouths and bodies are at odds and instructs the state to reject such people.[33] The *Lunyu* also insists that what is said must be enacted:

> 君子名之必可言也
> 言之必可行也
> What the exemplary person names must be speakable, what he/she says must be enactable.
> (*Lunyu* 13/1)

The *Xunzi* presents the matter as a contrast between the ease of talking while seated and the effort of rising to put speech into effect:

> 故坐而言之起而可設張而可施行
> Those who sit and talk should be able to stand and show that what they say can be established—that it can be enacted over a broad area.
> (*Xunzi* 23/45)

The *Mozi* uses a metaphor of two parts of a matching tally to specify how speech and action should be mutually aligned. Its tally metaphor makes speech and action the measure for one another:

> 若之二士者言相非而行相反與
> 當使若二士者言必信行必果使言行之合猶合
> 符節也 無言而不行也

> It is as if there are two scholars, each of whose speech denies that of the other and whose action opposes that of the other. Now, if you make it so that their speech has to be trustworthy and their action has to produce results, that is, make their speech and actions unified, like unifying parts of a tally, then there would be no speech that is not enacted.
> (*Mozi* 16/29)

This metaphor indicates that speech and action will only serve as a basis for knowledge if they match like two parts of a tally. The character of human beings consists in their speech and action; hence understanding them depends upon observance of their speech and action. Both of these elements are decisive in creating character, but in isolation they are not necessarily reliable. In particular, because speech can exceed action, one must ensure that the two coincide.

The need to make speech and action tally amounts to matching the senses of hearing and seeing. This notion of tallying hearing and seeing evokes the verifying knowledge, referred to in the *Zhengming* chapter of the *Xunzi*. While the *Zhengming* does not articulate what "verification" involves, it seems likely that it entails comparing and tallying. My hypothesis is that verifying knowledge amounts to tallying what is heard by the ears with what is seen by the eyes. (The reasons for this are given in Chapter 3.) Once the heartmind tallies the ears and eyes, it produces speech, which, according to the *Zhengming* merits being called knowing. (However, the *Zhengming* chapter does not mention that the heartmind also produces action.) In any case, even without the corroboration from the *Zhengming*, it seems undeniable that hearing and seeing play a far more important role in knowing than the other senses, and that part of their role depends upon the two senses matching one another.

Additional Evidence of Aural/Visual Pairing

The persistence of aural and visual pairs even in contexts where one or the other element does not seem to fit provides further evidence of their significance. The aural and visual pairing is apparent in the way the *Zhuangzi* character, Ziqi of Nanguo, queries his attendant about his knowledge of the pipes of earth:

> 夫大塊噫氣其名為風...
> 而獨不聞之翏翏乎...
> 而獨不見之調調之刁刁乎
> The great clump of earth blows out *qi* whose name is "wind"...have you alone not *heard* the hubbub!...have you alone not *seen* how the stirring quivers!
> (*Zhuangzi* 2/4–8, emphasis added)

Hence, even when asking about something predominantly aural—the "pipes" of earth—the pattern demands a balance with the visual. So too, when describing an eye, the *Mencius* (consciously or not) takes the rather unnecessary step of tacking on an assertion that speech also reveals what goes on within the breast. The *Mencius* says the pupil of the eye is bright or dull in accordance with the center of the chest being correct or not:

> 存乎人者莫良於眸子
> 眸子不能掩其惡
> 胸中正則眸子瞭焉
> 胸中不正則眸子眊焉
> 聽其言觀其眸子人焉廋哉
> Within the person, there's nothing more wonderful than the pupil of the eye. The pupil cannot cover a person's badness. If within the breast things are aligned, then the pupil is clear. If within the breast things are not aligned, then the pupil is dull. *Listen to a person's speech* and look

> at his/her pupils:[34] how can the person be concealed? (*Mencius* 4A16, emphasis added.)

Like this case in the *Mencius* that includes the aural where it is not necessary, a case in the *Mozi* also includes the aural without reason. In a description of the sage's clothing, it notes pointlessly that their clothes do not dazzle the ears:

> 聖王之為衣服適身體和肌膚而足矣
> 非榮耳目而觀愚民也
> The sages made their clothes just to suit their bodies, not for dazzling ears and eyes or showing stupid people. (*Mozi* 6/12)

Thus, there are repeated occurrences of the ears and eyes in contexts where one sense alone would suffice. These occurrences point to not only the importance of the two senses but the importance of their pairing. The desired and known things of the world are aural or visual in nature, and they also form a complement to one another.

Conclusions

In their prominent role in these texts, the senses of hearing and sight sometimes substitute for the senses as a whole. But it seems that hearing and seeing do quite a bit more than stand in for the other senses. In and of themselves, they seem to indicate knowledge of the world and the power to control it.

Even more significantly, a surprising variety of things that are desired and known conform to either being heard or being seen. In these texts, aurality and visuality seem to represent a very basic way in which the universe is divided. Both human beings and things tend to manifest themselves as partly aural and partly visual, and the two form a pair of complementary parts. While many of the references to hearing and seeing do not mention that they should match, the pairing itself implicitly suggests they should. What the ear hears should tally with what the eye sees, and if it does not, knowledge is not possible.

Chapter 3: The Heartmind's Relation to the Senses

While the heartmind is superior to the senses in certain ways, much of its role is not too different from that of the senses. The *Mencius* and the *Xunzi* are careful to point out that the heartmind is the ruler of the other senses. But in the passages that deal with the functions of the heartmind and the senses, the heartmind's similarity to the other senses is often striking. The very notion of the "heartmind"—as one function that both emotes and thinks—makes an important point in this regard: its thinking and feeling cannot be disengaged from one another. This chapter aims to situate this thinking/feeling function in terms of its relation to sensing. If the heartmind feels as well as thinks, does it also sense? My contention is that the heartmind is, if not a sense itself, then very closely related to them. To make this argument, this chapter will examine various traits ascribed to the heartmind, ranging from the simple act of discrimination to what the *Zhengming* chapter of the *Xunzi* calls verifying knowledge. Afterwards, it will counterbalance claims about the heartmind's superiority with a presentation of its similarities to the other senses. The fragmented evidence in these texts cannot provide a definitive conclusion that the heartmind is a sense, but it does undermine the view that the heartmind is *radically* distinct from the senses.

Activities of the Heartmind

Warring States philosophical texts ascribe only a handful of activities to the heartmind, one of the most basic of which seems to be "discriminating" or "distinguishing." The description of the heartmind in the *Zhengming* says that, like the senses, the heartmind makes discriminations. Although discriminating is not unique to the heartmind, it is still a significant part of the heartmind's function. The *Mozi* cites the heartmind's distinguishing as the defining feature of an intelligent person:

> 慧者心辯而不繁説
> 多力而不伐功
> Intelligent people's heartminds distinguish, but they do not speak in complex ways.
> They have much strength, but they do not boast of their deeds.
> (*Mozi* 2/12–13)

While the *Mozi* highlights the importance of the heartmind's distinguishing, the *Zhengming* specifies which categories it distinguishes:

> 説故喜怒哀樂愛惡欲以心異
> Speech and causes, happiness and anger, sadness and joy, loves, hates, and desires are differentiated by the heartmind.
> (*Xunzi* 22/19)

If we ignore the first two items, this looks like a series of emotions. But because "speech" and "causes" are included, we might say this is a group of "categories," strongly influenced by emotions. Drawing distinctions between these categories is one of the heartmind's basic operations.

The heartmind's pondering seems to build upon its distinguishing.[1] The items distinguished by the heartmind in the *Zhengming* bear a significant resemblance to what the *Xunzi* elsewhere calls the *qing* (conditions? dispositions?).[2] These *qing* are what the *Xunzi* uses to explain the heartmind's pondering. After introducing the notion of a person's nature or "what he/she is born with," the *Xunzi* says,

性之好惡喜怒哀樂謂之情
情然而心為之擇謂之慮
The nature's love, hatred, pleasure, anger, sadness, and happiness: [we] call this *qing* [condition? disposition?].
Given that the *qing* is like this, the heartmind's acting upon this and selecting: [we] call this pondering.
(*Xunzi* 22/3)

The passage implies that pondering amounts to selecting. The notion that pondering consists in selection is reinforced by the use of similar characters (*ze* 擇 and *qu* 取) to describe the heartmind's actions. A passage from the *Zhuangzi* seems to refer to the heartmind's "self-selection":

夫隨其成心而師之
誰獨且無師乎
奚必知代而心自取者有之
愚者與有焉
But if you accord with your completed heartmind and make it your authority, who is without such an authority?
Why should it be someone who knows alternations and whose heartmind selects by itself who has such an authority? A stupid person has one also.
(*Zhuangzi* 2/21–22)

The emphasis on *self* selections seems to recur in the expression of the heartmind's independence, as described in the *Xunzi*.[3] Once again, that text speaks in the same breath of *qing* and the heartmind's selections:

心容其擇也無禁必自見
其物也雜博
其情之至也不貳
Of the heartmind's manner, its selections cannot be prohibited. It must see by itself. Though things may be

> varied and extensive, the arrival at its *qing* [conditions? dispositions?] will not be divided.
> (*Xunzi* 21/46–47)

Given the *Xunzi* 22/3 reference (above) to selecting *qing*, I take this portrait of the heartmind's independence to concern selection of *qing*. No matter how varied the things confronting it, the heartmind will "see by itself" (more on this image below). It does so by directly selecting *qing* (that is, either selecting a "condition" from among the things or selecting a "disposition" in response to the things). In light of these repeated references to selections, we may infer that the description of pondering as selecting among *qing* is no idle quirk on the part of one author. In these texts, it seems that the heartmind ponders by selecting among the categories that it discriminates.

Through a process that the texts describe as "seeking" (*qui* 求) and "obtaining" (*de* 得), this pondering leads to knowing. Both the *Xunzi* and the corrupted chapters of the *Mozi*, known as the "Neo-Mohist Canons," compare the heartmind's pondering to an eye's seeking for a needle. The *Xunzi* passage reads,

> 今夫亡箴者終日求之而不得
> 其得之非目益明也
> 眸而見之也心之於慮亦然
> Now when it is a case of a needle being lost, one can seek all day and not find it. Finding it is not a matter of the eye gaining additional clarity. [One uses one's] pupil and sees it. The heartmind's pondering is also like this.[4]
> (*Xunzi* 27/64–65)

If A. C. Graham's reconstruction of the Neo-Mohist Canons is successful enough to be used as evidence, Canon A 4 repeats the analogy, but adds that pondering does not necessarily obtain what it looks for.[5]

> A 4 慮求也
> (慮)〔慮〕也者以其知有求也而不必得之(若睨)
> A 4 To ponder is to seek.
> (Ponder) "Ponder": by means of one's knowing one seeks something, but does not necessarily obtain it. (Like peering).
> (Graham, *Later Mohist Logic, Ethics and Science,* 266, translation modified)

Thus, pondering is like seeking, but it may not find what it seeks. This notion that the heartmind seeks to obtain something may be illuminated by another aspect of the *Xunzi*. The *Xunzi* compares the difference between pondering and knowing to the difference between looking and seeing. That is, it presents a sequence that parallels seeing without looking to knowing without pondering:

> 不視而見不聽而聰不言而信不慮而知
> [The gentleman] does not look yet sees; does not listen yet hears; does not speak yet is trusted; does not ponder yet knows.
> (*Xunzi* 24/2)

Working from this analogy, we might say that the difference between looking and seeing is that looking does not necessarily obtain what it seeks. (For example, the *Xunzi* mentions that a blind person can "look" at the stars, but s/he cannot see them.)[6] Applying this to the heartmind, it seems that two of the heartmind's activities—pondering and knowing—relate to one another as seeking relates to obtaining. *Mencius* 6A15 (quoted below) says as much. The heartmind differs from the senses because of the fact that it thinks; and because it thinks, it obtains something.[7] Thus, the heartmind's pondering is a kind of seeking, and knowing means getting what it seeks.

The idea that the heartmind's knowing amounts to getting what it seeks evokes the ambiguity of its being both heart and mind. Seeking introduces an element of desire to these descriptions of the heartmind's knowing. It indicates desire insofar as it presupposes a desire to meet a goal. The relation of seeking to desire is especially close in these texts, where desires are very often described in terms of the character *qui* 求 (seek). For instance, the *Xunzi* explains the nature of desire in terms of seeking.[8] It says things like,

> 人生而有欲欲而不得則不能無求
> Once people are born, they have desires. And once there are desires that are not met, they cannot but seek to meet them.
> (*Xunzi* 19/1)

> 欲不待可得而求者
> Desires are such that they seek without waiting for what can be obtained.
> (*Xunzi* 22/57)

Portraying the heartmind as seeking means the heartmind's pondering is motivated by desire, and its knowing is getting what it desires. Thus, not only do the *qing* that the heartmind selects in its pondering resemble a catalogue of emotions, but the motivation to select among such emotions may be as compulsive as these impatient desires. This, too, characterizes the function as both heart and mind.

"Verifying Knowledge" in the Zhengming

In addition to knowing, the heartmind has the capacity for verifying knowing, according to the *Zhengming* chapter of the *Xunzi*. (The term does not appear elsewhere in these texts.) Before attempting to identify what the heartmind's verifying knowledge is, it is worth articulating what it is not. The *Zhengming* suggests that it is not a transcendent function that steps in to interpret sensations by means of names or judgments. In other words, just as notions of "perception" and "sensation" do not apply to sense discrimination in these texts, they also do not apply to the heartmind.

The depiction of sense discrimination must be read in light of the *Zhengming* chapter as a whole. The *Zhengming* professes to have a central aim: to show what the sages would need to investigate in order to make *new* names. The *Zhengming* does not try to describe an imaginary state (of a group or an individual) prior to the existence of speech and names. For its project of showing what is needed for new names, the *Xunzi* points out three agendas and addresses each in turn. The sages should consider (1) the "purpose of names" 所 為 有 名, (2) "what we rely on for distinguishing the same and the different" 所 緣 有 同 異, and (3) the "pivot for regulating names" 制 名 之 樞 要. In this three-part sequence, the sages' naming takes place in the first section and culminates in the third section, neither of which describes knowing. Verifying knowledge and what I call sensory knowledge only appear in the second section. This means that the *Zhengming*'s interest in the application of names to things has much to do with the *purpose* and *regulation* of names and only indirectly relates to knowledge based on sense discrimination. Moreover, it means that naming occurs in the *Zhengming*'s project from the very beginning. The sequence in the structure of the *Zhengming* does not present naming as something that can only occur after sense discrimination. Although it is true that the heartmind does have a special function in the *Zhengming*'s description of sense discrimination, its job is not to name or interpret data. Speech and interpretation already appear in the process of sense discrimination before the heartmind begins its special function.

The role of speech in the *Zhengming* is complex. The *Zhengming* mentions the ears' discrimination of sounds (*sheng* 聲)—a term that in some cases can indicate voices or speech.[9] The

Zhengming then places the heartmind's discrimination of speech, or spoken explanations (*shuo* 說), at the very same level:[10]

> 聲音清濁調竽奇聲以耳異....
> 說故喜怒哀樂愛惡欲以心異
> Sounds and tones, clear and muddy, modes and harmony, and strange sounds are differentiated by the ear....
> Speech and causes, happiness and anger, sadness and joy, loves, hates, and desires are differentiated by the heartmind.[11]
> (*Xunzi* 22/17–19)

Thus, speech is an aspect differentiated by the heartmind, as sound is differentiated by the ears. If I am correct that there is such a thing as sensory knowing, these differentiations of sound and speech seem to belong in that category.

Speech also plays an additional role in verifying knowledge—the special form of knowing attributed to the heartmind, working in tandem with the ears and eyes. But speech does not *name* things in this role. On the contrary, the passage simply notes that speech is necessary for *confirming* knowledge:

> 然而徵知必將待天官當簿其類
> 然後可也
> 五官簿之而不知心徵之而無說
> 則人莫不然謂之不知
> However, verifying must await the heavenly officers' meeting and recording their kinds in order to be possible. If the five officers record them without knowing, or if the heartmind verifies without speaking, then people will not fail to pronounce it "not knowing."[12]
> (*Xunzi* 22/19–21)

The passage does not elaborate on what it is about speech that permits the attribution of knowledge. At this point, the discussion of knowledge of sense discrimination ends. After the discussion of knowing, the second section very clearly comes to a close with the announcement that, "It is *this* that causes sameness and difference."

Not until the beginning of the last section does the *Xunzi* finally state that these (already known) distinctions between same and different should be followed and *named*—rendering similar the similar and different the different. In other words, the naming referred to in the first section's description of the "purpose of names" is not reintroduced in the second section's description of how discriminations are known by the senses and the heartmind, and verified by the heartmind. The final section concerning regulating names is where the same and different are named. Two things show that this naming of sameness and difference is not like interpreting uninterpreted sense data. First, as argued earlier, the differences are already imbued with meaning. Second, verifying is not a process of naming. The *Xunzi* does not explain how the heartmind progresses from the verifying knowing of the second section, which already requires speech (*shuo* 說), to the third section's naming the same and the different. However, the fact that naming only appears in the third section shows that verifying knowing is not the heartmind using its speech to name unnamed sense products.

Thus, the ears' discriminating sound and the heartmind's discriminating speech, as well as the heartmind's verifying knowledge, all occur *prior to decreeing names* (*ming* 命),[13] which does not reappear until the third section, the "pivot for regulating names." Hence, whatever verifying knowledge is, it is not a process whereby the heartmind names.

"Verifying Knowledge" outside the Zhengming

Although the term verifying knowledge only appears in the *Zhengming* chapter of the *Xunzi*, the idea may extend outside of that chapter. *Xunzi* 21/34–39 consists of a long description of the heartmind's knowledge, but aside from the claim that knowledge requires sameness and difference, nothing in the passage reflects the *Zhengming*'s discussion of verifying knowledge.[14] However, hints of something like verification seem present in other places. Some other activities ascribed to the heartmind would seem to be helpful for verification. For example, in *Mencius* 6A9, the heartmind "supposes," and in the *Xunzi* 21/33, the heartmind "endorses" something. Furthermore, the *Mozi* refers to the heartmind's failure to examine knowledge in a way that suggests it possesses the capacity to examine.[15] All of these actions—supposing, endorsing, and examining—may be likely to contribute to verification, but do not approximate the act of verifying itself.

My hypothesis is that the reference to the heartmind's tallying in the *Zhuangzi* is the closest thing to verification. The *Zhuangzi* implies that tallying is characteristic of the ordinary use of the heartmind. In the context of identifying the limitations of ordinary functions, the *Zhuangzi* comments that listening stops at the ears. Then it adds,

> ...心止於符
> ...the heartmind stops at tallying.
> (*Zhuangzi* 4/27)

In early Chinese history, tallies consisted of two sticks with matched notches. These were widely used as tokens of agreement—the carving on the tally being split in two when the tally was broken, and each half serving as proof of a promise.[16] While "supposing," "endorsing," and "examining" may all be useful for the purpose of verifying something, only "tallying" seems able to accomplish that purpose.

Other references to tallying in these texts provide support for the case that tallying might be what the *Zhengming* calls verifying knowledge. As this passage from the *Xunzi* implies, tallies derive their value from their ability to justify trust:

> 合符節別契券者所以為信也
> Uniting the halves of tallies and tokens and separating contracts and deeds are the reason for trust.
> (*Xunzi* 12/7)

The trust invested in a tally helps explain why the *Xunzi* characterizes creating strange names as a crime comparable to disrupting tallies (and other standards of measure). Speaking of those who interfere with correct names, the *Xunzi* says,

> 其罪猶為符節度量之罪也
> 故其民莫敢託為奇辭以亂正名
> Their crime is [treated] like those who violate tallies or weights and measures.
> Hence, [the true ruler's] people do not dare to make up strange phrases and disorder correct names.
> (*Xunzi* 22/8–9)

The connection of tallies with naming here is not arbitrary. Not only the allusion to trust, but also the mention of names is a reminder that what tallies accomplish in one sphere, correlating speech with action accomplishes in another. In other words, what makes trust possible in human relations (according to these texts) is speech that coincides with behavior, like two parts of a tally. Indeed, this is the metaphor the *Xunzi* uses:

> 凡論者貴其有辨合有符驗
> 故坐而言之起而可設
> 張而可施行
> In terms of those who analyze things, there is value in discrimination and matching, as well as tallying and confirming. Those who sit and talk should be able to stand and show that what they say can be established—that it can be enacted over a broad area.
> (*Xunzi* 23/44–45)

An even more explicit metaphor for matching speech with action like two parts of a tally appears in *Mozi* 16/29 (quoted in full in Chapter 2). This repeated use of a trustworthy tally as a metaphor for enacting speech sheds light on the *Zhuangzi*'s comment about the heartmind's tallying. The reader may recall that the *Zhengming* specifies that the heartmind uses the ears and eyes for verifying knowledge.[17] Thus, the evidence indicates four things: (1) that one of the heartmind's functions is tallying, (2) that speech and action need to be tallied, (3) that speech is heard and action is seen, and (4) that the heartmind verifies through the ears and eyes. In combination, this evidence points to the conclusion that the heartmind verifies by tallying the senses of hearing and vision.

The Heartmind's Status in Relation to the Senses

As mentioned in the beginning of the chapter, by virtue of some of its activities, the heartmind is presented as superior to the other senses in these texts. The consensus seems to be that, ordinarily, the heartmind controls the other parts of the person. The *Xunzi* says the heartmind is the ruler of the form.[18] It also notes that the heartmind governs the other senses, ordering the five officers from the center, where it is positioned:

> 心居中虛以治五官
> The heartmind dwells in the central emptiness, in order to govern the five officers.
> (*Xunzi* 17/12)

The *Mencius* contrasts the heartmind to the ears and eyes, calling the former the great part of a person and the latter the petty part. According to the *Mencius*, one should follow the heartmind, both because it is greater and because it is sent from heaven.[19] One should not let the ears and eyes undermine the heartmind's office:

> 耳目之官不思而蔽於物物交物則引之而已矣
> 心之官則思思則得之不思則不得也
> 此天之所與我者
> 先立乎其大者則其小者不能奪也
> Thinking is not the office of the eyes and ears, and they are clouded by things. Things interact with things, and pull them astray. That is all. The office of the heartmind is thinking. It thinks, and thus it obtains. If it does not think, then it does not obtain. This is what heaven has given me. If you first take your stand upon the great part, then the small part cannot take it away.
> (*Mencius* 6A15)

As the passage points out, the heartmind's ability to think gives it more self-control than the ears and eyes in the face of the things that tug at it. The *Zhuangzi* also recognizes that the heartmind is characteristically the master (although the *Zhuangzi* disagrees about the wisdom of putting the heartmind in control). One of the *Zhuangzi*'s characters criticizes someone for using his heartmind as his teacher (猶師心者也) in a way that indicates that generally the heartmind occupies the position of authority (*Zhuangzi* 4/24). Leadership is a capacity that the other senses do not seem to have, hence, the heartmind is superior in this respect.

The heartmind has the additional superior feature of helping the other senses to function. The *Xunzi* claims that, unless the heartmind is employed, hearing or seeing will not occur:

> 心不使焉則白黑在前而不見
> 雷鼓在側而耳不聞況於使者乎
> If the heartmind is not being applied to it, then black and white may be right before one's eyes and not be seen; thunder or drums may be at one's side and one's ears will not hear them. How much more so with one whose heartmind is occupied by something![20]
> (*Xunzi* 21/4–5)

In the *Zhengming*, the *Xunzi* repeats this claim, saying that, because of the heartmind's verifying knowing, it is possible to use the ears to know sounds and the eyes to know forms.[21] In addition to this assistance in knowing, the heartmind also seems to have a capacity to substitute for the senses, which the *Xunzi* claims the senses do not have[22] (more on this below). In its assistance to the other senses, as well as substitution for them, the heartmind manifests superiority and control.

Similarities Between the Heartmind and the (Other) Senses

Nevertheless, there are many reasons to think that the heartmind is like a sense, not the least of which is the fact that sensory lists often include the heartmind. The *Xunzi*, which is the most adamant about the heartmind's leadership, repeatedly lists the heartmind as one of the five senses. In some cases, there seems to be no discernible distinction between the heartmind and the rest of the senses.[23] For example, in the *Xunzi* 11/46–47 listing of what the senses desire, no changes in the rhetorical pattern serve to isolate the heartmind from the other senses (see Chapter 1). A similar kind of list of human *qing* includes the heartmind but omits the nose and adds the form and body. In a discussion of the role of the emperor, the *Xunzi* says that his circumstances combine all human desires:

> 故人之情
> 口好味而臭味莫美焉
> 耳好聲而聲樂莫大焉
> 目好色而文章致繁婦女莫眾焉
> 形體好佚而安重閒靜莫愉焉
> 心好利而穀祿莫厚焉
> Thus, the human *qing* [condition? disposition?] is such that the mouth is fond of tastes, yet no fragrant flavors are

> more beautiful [than what the emperor has]; the ear is fond of sounds, yet no sounds of music are more grand; the eye is fond of color, yet no ornaments or patterns extend more completely, nor are women more numerous; the form and limbs are fond of ease, yet no peace or weightiness, nor period of quietude is more pleasant; the heartmind is fond of profit, yet no payment or salary is more substantial.
> (*Xunzi* 11/78–80)

One might object that in both these examples the heartmind appears at the end of the list—a location that might alone serve to distinguish it from the other senses. But the heartmind does not always appear as the culmination of the list (see *Xunzi* 23/25–26 on page 19). Similarly, an example from the *Laozi* includes the heartmind in the midst of what appear to be sensory lists. The case from the *Laozi* manages to find one desired "object" that motivates the heartmind in the same way that, for example, tastes motivate the mouth. (Interestingly, it decides upon speedy horses, which also inspire desire in *Mozi* 36/18, *Mencius* 1B1, and *Zhuangzi* 2/81.)

> 五色使人目盲
> 馳騁田臘使人心發狂
> 難得之貨使人之行仿
> 五味使人之口爽
> 五音使人之耳聾
> The five colors cause people's eyes to go blind. Riding and hunting cause people's heartminds to go crazy. Goods that are hard to obtain cause people's actions to be obstructed; the five colors cause people's mouths to miss the mark. The five tones cause people's ears to go deaf.[24]
> (*Laozi* 12)

Once again, the subject seems to be the sensory desires, and in this regard, the heartmind seems very much like a sense.[25] Hence, insofar as it desires, the heartmind does not appear to be too different from the other senses.

Moreover, the heartmind's ability to substitute for the other senses renders it similar to the senses, even as it serves to mark its superiority. According to *Xunzi* 21/46–47 (above) the heartmind can see for itself. While this may sound like an insignificant metaphor, the *Xunzi* also mentions the heartmind's speaking and listening:

> 以仁心說以學心聽以公心辨
> Use a humane heartmind to speak; use a learned heartmind to listen; use a fair heartmind to discriminate.
> (*Xunzi* 22/45–46)

The heartmind's ability to listen appears in the *Zhuangzi* as well, as if it were an advance over ordinary listening with the ears:

> 無聽之以耳而聽之以心
> Do not listen with the ear, but listen with the heartmind.
> (*Zhuangzi* 4/27)

The heartmind's capacity to speak is also noted more than once. In addition to *Xunzi* 22/45, it appears in the *Zhengming* and the *Mencius*. The *Zhengming* implies that the heartmind has the capacity to speak, by saying that if it does not speak, then no one will credit it with knowing.[26] The *Mencius* actually cites the heartmind's speech:

> 其心曰是何足與言仁義也云爾
> Their heartminds say, "This person is not fit to speak with about humaneness and righteousness."
> (*Mencius* 2B2)

Thus, the heartmind sees, listens, and speaks in a variety of contexts. Even if these are all metaphors—cloaking no beliefs that the heartmind has the capacity to substitute for the other senses—these passages paint the heartmind as a physically interactive function. A heartmind that is said to see, listen, and speak cannot seem radically divorced from the senses.

Other senses serve as analogies for the heartmind, which contributes to the sense that there are similarities between them. For example, the *Xunzi* mentions an unnamed thinker, who believes the heartmind's goodness inheres in it like good eyesight inheres in the eye:

> 所謂性善者不離其朴而美之不離其資而利之也
> 使夫資朴之於美心意之於善
> 若夫可以見之明不離目
> 可以聽之聰不離耳
> 故曰目明而耳聰也
>
> The so-called view that "[human] nature is good" takes its [the nature's] failure to leave its plain state as beauty and its failure to separate from its original character as beneficial. Such a view compares the plain state's relation to beauty, as well as the intent of the heartmind's relation to goodness, to the way brightness of ocular capacity does not leave the eyes and keenness of aural capacity does not leave the ears, (whence comes the saying "bright eye and keen ear").
> (*Xunzi* 23/15–17)

The view described here finds fault with the deleterious effects of distance in time and space. This view objects to leaving the heartmind's original state on the same principle that brightness and keenness do not venture far from the eyes and ears.[27] The point seems to be that the pinnacle of goodness lies in remaining in the heartmind's original state, for the same reason that the eyes and ears function best when things are close to them (either in space or time). The analogy in the *Mencius* is a bit more straightforward.

The *Mencius* notes that, just as the sages set the standards of the mouth and eyes, so too they set the standards for the heartmind:

> 口之於味也有同耆焉
> 耳之於聲也有同聽焉
> 目之於色也有同美焉
> 至於心獨無所同然乎....
> 故理義之悅我心猶芻豢之悅我口
>
> In the relation of mouths to taste, there is similarity in what they relish. In the relation of ears to sounds, there is similarity in what they listen to. In the relation of eyes to color, there is similarity in what they find beauty in. As for the heartmind, does it alone lack similarities in what it approves of?...Therefore, the way pattern and righteousness please my heartmind is like the way the flesh of animals pleases my mouth.
> (*Mencius* 6A7)

According to these two analogies, the heartmind and the senses have certain things in common—they function on the same principles regarding space and time, and they share the tendency to prefer similar things. The fact that the senses serve as analogies for the heartmind makes it unlikely that they are radically different in nature.

The metaphor of the heartmind as a mirror does not explicitly compare the heartmind to the senses, but it still manages to highlight their similarities. These texts treat a pan of water as a potential standard of measure. They say the heartmind is like a pan of water, insofar as it reflects what passes before it. They use the water-mirror metaphor to emphasize, not representation, but the ability to respond to changing stimulation. As the *Zhuangzi* puts it,

> 至人之用心若鏡不將不迎
> 應而不藏故能勝物而不傷

> People of achievement use the heartmind like a mirror. They do not escort or welcome. They respond, but do not store. Therefore, they are able to conquer things and not be harmed.
> (*Zhuangzi* 7/32)

The *Zhuangzi* passage notes that for a mirror to be effective, it cannot escort what has come or welcome what will come. Such storing inhibits its ability to respond. The reference to response suggests stimulation, and indeed, the heartmind can be stimulated. A character in the *Zhuangzi* objects to having his heartmind stimulated by an offer of power:

> 汝又何帠以治天下感予之心為
> What are you doing stimulating my heartmind with the prospect of ruling the world?
> (*Zhuangzi* 7/10)

Thus, the mirroring heartmind operates on the same principle of stimulus and response that characterizes the operation of the senses.[28]

The mirror metaphor also shows that, in addition to being stimulated, the heartmind resembles the senses in being enticed by things. Whereas the *Zhuangzi* juxtaposes the heartmind's storage to its response, the *Xunzi* makes a similar point via an opposition between storage and emptiness. The *Xunzi* says that the heartmind can store its aims as long as it remains empty—that is, as long as they do not interfere with its receptiveness:

> 人生而有知知而有志志也者臧也
> 然而有所謂虛
> 不以所已臧害所將受謂之虛
> Once people are born, there is knowledge, once there is knowledge, there is the heartmind's aims. The heartmind's aims are its storing. And yet the heartmind has what is

> called emptiness. Not letting what has been stored damage what is to be received is called emptiness.
> (*Xunzi* 21/36–37)

The passage says the storage in the heartmind pertains to its aims or the directions in which it heads.[29] The implication seems to be that repeated aims are stored in the heartmind, perhaps in the form of habits. While this passage suggests that the heartmind should not let its aims interfere with its receptiveness, the *Xunzi*'s own mirror metaphor indicates that its success in this regard is rare. It implies that the mirror of the heartmind is easily disrupted by the passing of the wind, rendering it unable to reflect.[30] Using the same character from *Mencius* 6A15 to describe how things tug (*yin* 引) at the senses, the *Xunzi* goes on to assert that the heartmind's mirror is vulnerable to the enticement of things:

> 小物引之則其正外易
> 其心內傾則不足以決庶理矣
> If small things pull it, then its correct exterior alters and the heartmind's interior overturns. Then it is not sufficient to settle various patterns.
> (*Xunzi* 21/57–58)

Thus, contrary to the claim in *Xunzi* 21/44–46, the heartmind is not unlike the senses in being pulled by things. The mirror metaphor betrays the resemblance: like the senses, the heartmind only functions properly when the undue influence of external things does not disrupt it.

In the course of its interaction with things, parts of the heartmind seem to move from the inside to the outside. The *Mencius* describes the heartmind in terms of exiting, as well as entering. At one time, Mencius considers a saying of Confucius and determines that it applies to the heartmind:

> 操則存舍則亡出入無時莫知其鄉
> 惟心之謂與
> "Hold it and it is preserved, cast it off and it is lost.
> Its entrances and exits lack regular timing, and no one knows its place." Isn't this said of the heartmind?
> (*Mencius* 6A8)

Although the passage does not specify what enters and exits, it certainly affirms that entering and exiting are features of the heartmind. Thus things exit from the heartmind, as well as entering it.

A variety of things can emerge from the heartmind. The *Xunzi* mentions that shapes (or "forms") leave the heartmind:

> 異形離心交喻異物
> 名實玄紐貴賤不明同異不別
> If heterodox [different] forms leave the heartmind, encountering and illuminating heterodox [different] things, then name and filling will be mysterious and knotted, noble and base will not be clear, same and different will not be distinguished.[31]
> (*Xunzi* 22/13)

To understand the concern that strange forms might leave the heartmind, it may help to consider a passage from the *Zhuangzi* that speaks of things being bound to the heartmind:

> 天下有大戒二
> 其一命也其一義也
> 子之愛親命也不可解於心
> The world has two great commandments. One is ordained and the other is duty. A child's love for its parents is ordained. It cannot be unbound from the heartmind.
> (*Zhuangzi* 4/39–40)

In light of the possibility that things can be let loose from the heartmind, the *Xunzi* passage seems to say that odd items should not be allowed to escape the heartmind and cause chaos in their encounters with things.

Peace is also something that can escape or be "emitted" (*chu* 出) from the heartmind, according to the *Zhuangzi*.[32] In preparation for contact with a dangerous person, one of *Zhuangzi*'s characters suggests rectifying the body. He elaborates on this as wanting the form to approach without entering and wanting the heartmind to have peace without emitting:

> 正女身也哉
> 形莫若就心莫若和
> 雖然之二者有患
> 就不欲入和不欲出
> 形就而入且為顛為滅為崩為蹶
> 心和而出且為聲為名為妖為孽
>
> **Align your body! In form, there is nothing like the approach. In the heartmind, there is nothing like peace. However, these two have difficulties. With approaching, you don't want to enter. With peace, you don't want to emit. If the form approaches and enters, then there will be overturning, disaster, collapse, and stumbling. If the heartmind has peace but emits it, then there will be sound, fame, uncanny events, and retribution.[33]**
> **(*Zhuangzi* 4/56–58)**

In this balancing act of entering and exiting, the *Zhuangzi* says it is dangerous to allow peace to exit from the heartmind.

The *Mencius* seems to posit other things emerging from the heartmind. The *Mencius* states explicitly that something rooted in the heartmind will appear in the visual expression:

> 根於心其生色也
> 睟然見於面

> [These are] rooted in the heartmind and born in the complexion. They are manifest agreeably in the face. (*Mencius* 7A21)

The *Mencius* also refers to speech being "instigated in" (*zuo yu* 作於) the heartmind. When it justifies why Mencius engages in debates with nonorthodox thinkers, the text refers to something as being instigated in the heartmind. The subject is slightly ambiguous, but Mencius is quoted as saying that he drives away their excessive phrases (speech) so that perverse speakers cannot instigate things. He then adds that what is instigated in the heartmind will subsequently obstruct affairs and governing:

> 距楊墨放淫辭邪說者不得作
> 作於其心害於其事作於其事害於其政
> I resist Yang and Mo, drive away their excessive expressions, so that perverse speakers do not instigate things. [Such] things that are instigated in the heartmind, obstruct in affairs. [Such] things that are instigated in affairs, obstruct in government.
> (*Mencius* 3B9)

The likelihood that speech is what is instigated in the heartmind is supported by another passage that says more or less the same thing about excessive phrases and obstructing governing. Here Mencius defends what he means by saying he "knows speech," and in this case seems to describe speech as "born in" (*sheng yu* 生於) the heartmind. Mencius appears to say that by knowing speech, he means inferring something about the source of the heterodox phrases (speech). The subject of the next clause is unclear, but it states that something is "born in" the heartmind that obstructs governing. Because Mencius was just speaking of the source of various illicit phrases, and is now speaking of something being born, it is likely that the subject is these phrases whose source he knows:

何謂知言曰詖辭知其所蔽
淫辭知其所陷邪辭知其所離
遁辭知其所窮
生於其心害於其政發於其政害於其事
"What does it mean to know speech?" Mencius replied, "From one-sided phrases, I know that from which they cloud. From excessive phrases, I know that from which they sink. From bad phrases, I know that from which they estrange; from evasive phrases, I know that from which they exhaust.
What is born in their heartminds obstructs in their governing; what issues from their governing obstructs in their affairs."
(*Mencius* 2A2)

Thus, in addition to causing facial expressions, the *Mencius* seems to say the heartmind causes speech to be instigated or born. While this is not as explicit as a term like "exit," it does hint at interaction (albeit indirect) between the heartmind and the exterior of the person. This may be what the *Zhuangzi* means by implying that inward channels of the eyes and ears can lead to expelling the heartmind's knowledge (see *Zhuangzi* 4/32–33, page 59). From this perspective, the heartmind's external vent depends upon its connection to the ears and eyes. In any case, the *Mencius* suggests that speech and visual expression "exit" from the heartmind. Thus, the heartmind is like the other senses insofar as it interacts with things.

Conclusions

While the heartmind may rule the senses, it is not unlike them. The heartmind's capacity to distinguish seems to be something it shares with the senses. If we take these analogies seriously, its pondering is comparable to the eye's looking. To some extent, even its knowing may be a feature that all of the senses share (as argued in Chapter 1). The *Xunzi* and the *Mencius* insist that the heartmind has more balance and self-control than the senses. But perhaps their claims implicitly admit that the difference is a matter of degrees. Only the heartmind's verifying knowledge seems qualitatively different from anything performed by the senses. If I am right that this verifying corresponds to the heartmind's tallying things heard and seen, then there is a significant reason why the senses of hearing and seeing are featured so prominently in these texts.

The heartmind does have some capacity that permits it to rule over the senses. But this does not eliminate the possibility that the heartmind is a sense, or very much like a sense. In fact, it seems to be the proper consequence of the ruler analogy that the heartmind would be one of the senses. Rulers may be superior to their subjects in important ways, but even if they are descendants of ancestors in heaven, they are not a different species of being.

Chapter 4: Names and Their "Filling"

As noted in the Introduction, many sinologists describe the early Chinese cosmology in terms of an organismic process. Such a cosmos, they argue, has no room for eternally unchanging substances or realities. Instead of immutability, at best the cosmos offers constant patterns amidst change (epitomized by things like the seasons and the alternation of night and day). The regularity of patterns provides the basis for order, which seems to be the main concern of Warring States philosophical texts. Change is inevitable, but not disastrous—as long as there is regularity in the constant patterns of the cosmos. This chapter contributes evidence for that view of the early Chinese cosmos, by focusing on the implicit role of change in one central feature of the worldview expressed in these texts. That is, I will suggest that intimations of change are present in the use of the character *shi* 實, which is frequently translated as "substance" or "reality." *Shi* appears together with *ming* 名 (names) in a dyad that seems to refer to a very basic division of the world.[1] This chapter argues that there are two aspects of change associated with the use of the character *shi*: (1) The character is used to signify the product of a process (a "fruit"). (2) It is also used within an aural/visual pair. I contend that "names and *shi*" is an aural/visual pairing, like "speech and action" described in Chapter 2. As the partner term for names, *shi* is visual in nature, and insofar as vision correlates with action (as Chapter 2 argues), *shi* also indicates activity, and therefore change.

"Fruit" versus "Substance" and "Reality"

Translating the character *shi* as "substance" obscures its frequent association with notions of change. This sense of change can be highlighted by focusing on the connotations of the term's use as "fruit." Fruition is a matter of becoming full, in the sense of a seed, which grows by filling out its spatial boundaries.

Xu Shen's (c. 55–149) Han dictionary, the *Shuo wen jie zi*, clearly post-dates the Warring States period, but must be addressed because of its widespread influence.[2] The *Shuo wen* glosses *shi* as *fu* 富 "wealth." Indeed, *shi* 實 is composed of three parts—a "roof," as well as a "string" and "shells" (suggesting coins strung together). The *Shuo wen* gloss seems to encourage the idea that the constitution of the character *shi* consists of strings of coins filling up a house, hence seemingly indicating wealth as a storehouse of substances. However, in the composition of a character containing the element "roof," what is underneath the roof need not be something *inside of* that roof. *Fu* 富 itself is a graph composed of a "roof" and a "field," and, in addition to "wealth," its use has an extended connotation of "fullness." But it seems unlikely that this connotation refers to a field that is underneath a roof filling up a house like a container. The same point applies to *shi*. On this model, the *Shuo wen*'s suggestion that *shi* means "filling" is unlikely to refer to substances filling up a house. Instead, it may be related to *shi*'s function as "fruit." In the organic sense of the term, *shi* fills space by growing and expanding its contours.[3] (Similarly, *shi* and its opposite *xu* 虛—empty—may refer to a stomach, which changes shape as it moves from empty to full.)[4] In other words, the filling does not involve adding substance to a container that has a permanently fixed shape. The focus of filling in the use of the character *shi* is on the filling out of space, like a seed growing to fruition.

The *Zhengming* chapter of the *Xunzi* confirms this emphasis on the importance of spatial filling for understanding *shi*. When the *Xunzi* explains how *shi* can be counted, it says that if something has the same manner, but is different in spatial location, then, although it can be united, we should call it "two" *shi*. Thus, the relevant feature in counting *shi*—even if it has the same manner—seems to be how it fills space:

> 有異狀而同所者可別也
> 狀同而為異所者雖可合謂之二實

狀變而實無別而異者謂之化
有化而無別謂之一實
此事之所以稽實定數也
Things that have different shapes but occupy the same place can be separated. If the shape is the same, but the place is different, although they can be united, call them two *shi*. If the shape changes, but the *shi* has not been separated, although it is different, call it transformed. Things that transform without being separated, call them one *shi*. This process is how *shi* are investigated and numbers are determined.
(*Xunzi* 22/27–29)

Thus, whether or not a *shi* is divided determines whether to call it one *shi*. If there is transformation without division, the *Xunzi* calls it one *shi*. If by "division" the *Xunzi* means split into two, then again the emphasis seems to be on occupation of space. The criteria for being one *shi*, then, are that (1) it is not in two places and (2) it is not divided (perhaps again, by place). A *shi* can alter its manner and still be one *shi*, but if it fills different spaces, it becomes two *shi*. Hence the sense in which *shi* connotes fullness lies in how it fills space. Its solidity (or substantiality) is secondary—a byproduct of this filling.

Like the translation of *shi* as "substance," the translation of *shi* as "reality" also obscures the notion of change implicit in the use of the character. The term "reality" has a variety of uses in English that do not suit *shi*—particularly its use in opposition to illusion and nonexistence.[5] Moreover, while "reality" invariably connotes authenticity, such connotations are not bound to appear in the use of *shi*. This means, as I will argue below, that certain translations of *shi* as "reality" do not produce the most coherent interpretations of the texts.

Although things that are not *shi* are generally described as empty, emptiness is not unreality.[6] Even in the contexts where empty is associated with falsity (*jia* 假), emptiness is not a matter of illusion masking nonexistence. Rather, when something empty is false, it is because some potential is not being fulfilled. For example, the *Mozi* refers to emptiness and falseness as not being embodied, i.e., filled by the body:

> 君子之道貧則見廉
> 富則見義生則見愛死則見哀
> 四行者不可虛假反之身者也
> 藏於心者無以竭愛
> 動於身者無以竭恭
> 出於口者無以竭馴
>
> The way of noble people is such that, as to poverty, they are pure; as to wealth, they are righteous; as to life, they are loving; and as to death, they are sad. These four actions cannot be emptied and falsified in contrast to their bodies. There is nothing hidden in their heartminds that is not the utmost effort to love. There is nothing that moves from their bodies that is not the utmost effort to be respectful. There is nothing emitted from their mouths that is not the utmost effort to be mild.
> (*Mozi* 2/6–8)

In other words, these actions are empty when the heartmind, the body, and the mouth do not "ful-fill" them—indeed, fulfill them by manifesting them to the utmost point of exhaustion. Thus, emptiness is not unreal in the sense of being non-existent or illusory. The implication is that an empty action is like a dormant seed of potential that is not carried out.

An empty name provides an even clearer illustration of what emptiness connotes. Such a name is not illusory in the sense that it does not exist. The *Mozi* says that actions are the source of names (fame). An empty name is one that flows obscurely from a murky, untrustworthy original act:

原濁者流不清
行不信者名必耗
名不徒生而譽不自長
功成名遂名譽不可虛假
When the origin is muddy, the flow is not clear. When actions are not trustworthy, one's name/fame will certainly be exhausted. Names are not just born, praise does not grow on its own. When effort is achieved, one's name follows, and the name and praise cannot be empty and false.
(*Mozi* 2/11)

There is a contrast here between, on the one hand, the act of effortless birth and growth, and, on the other, the achievement of an effort. The contrast indicates that the emptiness or falseness of a name reflects that it did not originate in an act of striving. Such a name can be called "misleading," but it is not illusory in the sense that it is not really there.

Likewise, the *Mencius*'s explanation of *shi* in terms of beauty in no way hints at the subject of illusion. In the *Mencius*'s aesthetic evaluation, fulfillment and emptiness designate degrees of beauty, not degrees of existence. Someone asks Mencius what he means by the terms "good" and "trustworthy." Mencius answers,

可欲之謂善有諸己之謂信
充實之謂美充實而有光輝之謂大
What can be desired is called good, and having it within oneself is called trustworthy. What is full and *shi* [brought to fruition] is called beauty. What is full, *shi,* and brightly displayed is called greatness.
(*Mencius* 7B25)

In this passage, *shi* is something beautiful, insofar as it is completely manifest—it extends through its fullness and brightness of display. By contrast, emptiness would be something not fully manifest. Because the *Mencius* presents this contrast in terms of degrees of beauty, this too supports the interpretation that when emptiness connotes falsity, it is because of nonfulfillment, rather than illusion or nonexistence.

Like reality versus illusion, the opposition of authenticity versus inauthenticity can be misleading when applied to *shi*. In some circumstances, *shi* is interchangeable with the character *qing* 情, and seems to connote authenticity.[7] However, when contrasted to emptiness, *shi* is not always the more favored of the two, which makes it incongruous to view *shi* as authentic. For example, heaven's emptiness (or tenuousness) seems to contrast positively against the qualities of earth—that is, whereas the earth is heavy and damp, heaven is empty, warm, and bright.[8] Rather than rendering heaven less authentic, the greater tenuousness of heaven seems to be part of the overall superiority of the powers on high. The value of emptiness is also apparent in the *Xunzi*'s praise for the heartmind's emptiness, which provides the space that allows it to govern (*Xunzi* 17/12) and be receptive to new aims in spite of already stored aims (*Xunzi* 21/36–37). Thus, while in some contexts, the use of *shi* implies authenticity, in other contexts, emptiness possesses advantages that preclude viewing *shi* as the more authentic of the two.

The Mengsun Cai passage of the *Zhuangzi* illustrates the danger of insisting that *shi* is authentic. In this passage, "Confucius" (the mouthpiece of the *Zhuangzi*) praises the very people whom Yan Hui describes as lacking *shi*. Yan Hui asks,

> 孟孫才其母死
> 哭泣無涕中心不戚居喪不哀
> 無是三者以善處喪蓋魯國
> 固有無其實而得其名者乎
>
> When Mengsun Cai's mother died, his cries and wails lacked tears. His inner/central heartmind was not sad. While residing in mourning, he did not grieve. Though lacking these three things, his excellence at being in mourning

> covers the whole state of Lu. Are there indeed people who obtain a name for something without its *shi* [filling]? (*Zhuangzi* 6/75–76)

When answering this last question, Confucius does not deny that Mengsun has the name but lacks the *shi.* Yet, nonetheless, he praises him, saying that Mengsun has gone beyond knowledge and simply wails when another person wails. If we translate *shi* as "authenticity," then Confucius's answer seems to praise Mengsun for lacking in authenticity/reality. While Yan Hui does present Confucius with a puzzle, it is doubtful that the puzzle is quite so bizarre as this. Translating *shi* as "real" makes the passage say that emotions are genuine, while behavior is mere appearance. From this view, Mengsun Cai got the name *and* did the deed (mourned) but lacked the real, authentic emotion.

My contention is that such an interpretation is too quick to categorize certain things as actions and certain other things as emotions. The passage states that, in addition to sadness and grief, Mengsun lacked tears. Tears are not emotions. They might be counted as *expressions of* emotion, but according to that conception of emotion, so too would crying and wailing, with which Mengsun is credited.[9] Thus, on that view, Mengsun could not be said to lack emotions. Moreover, sadness is described as an action in *Mozi* 2/6–7, which opens the possibility that Mengsun (who is said to lack sadness) did not perform at least *one* relevant action. Indeed, perhaps there is no antithesis here between actions and emotions.

There is little reason to assume that, in these texts, emotions are something other than a type of action. If emotions are manifestations and expressions, then these too are actions. The alternative is to think that emotions are private entities/events that are located within hearts and minds and never manifest on the "outside." Certain translations of *Zhuangzi* 5/45–46 may mistakenly imply the view that emotions are privately located in the heartmind. When asked about "completed abilities," "Confucius" says:

> 死生存亡窮達貧富賢於不肖毀譽饑渴寒暑
> 是事之變命之行也
> 日夜相代乎前而知不能規乎其始者也
> 故不足以滑和不可入乎靈府使之和豫
> 通而不失於兑
> 使日夜無郤而與物為春
> 是接而生時於心者也是之謂才全
>
> Death and life, persistence and loss, exhaustion and achievement, poverty and wealth, competence and incompetence, slander and praise, hunger and thirst, cold and heat. These are the changes of events, the actions of *ming* [fate/ordainment/decree]. Day and night, they mutually alternate in front of us, and knowledge cannot measure their origins.
>
> Therefore they are not sufficient to disturb one's harmony. They cannot enter one's spiritual residence.
>
> To make it so that harmony and ease circulate, but are not lost in openings,[10] to make it so that, while night and day lack a break, together with things, one is like springtime, this is to greet [things] and to generate timeliness in the heartmind. This is called "completed abilities."
>
> (*Zhuangzi* 5/43–46)

Rather than a sealed storehouse, the *lingfu* (spiritual residence) image described here points to a place that permits open circulation. The references to generating timeliness and an ever-readiness to begin (like springtime) make the heartmind seem responsive and open as it "greets" things. Loss of peace and ease is avoided, not by sealing up a container, but by maintaining an equilibrium in the midst of inside/outside interaction.[11] Emotions of harmony and ease circulate (or interact, *tong* 通), while the heartmind greets things in a timely fashion. It is possible to envision a circulation of private entities/events inside a closed container, but it seems more likely that these emotions circulate inside and outside as manifestations and expressions.

In applying this notion of emotions as actions to the Mengsun passage, we might say that by lacking tears, sadness, and grief, Mengsun "lacked the *shi* " insofar as he did not *fully* perform the act of mourning. Perhaps Mengsun's mourning was not brought to fruition. Fruition requires development and completion. In that case—rather than singling out emotion as genuine, in contrast to actions as inauthentic—the point of the use of *shi* may be that Mengsun did not complete the *acts of feeling* necessary to fulfill the name "mourning." Thus, when Confucius praises Mengsun for wailing because another person wails, he is not praising him for lacking authentic and real emotions. On the contrary, he praises him for an act of feeling that he views as authentic, in spite of—or even perhaps because—it did not bring a name to fruition. Perhaps Mengsun and Confucius are liberated from the requirement of tallying name and *shi*. This may be what Confucius means by saying that Mengsun has gone beyond knowledge, (that is, as I argue below, like matching speech and action, matching names and *shi* may be constitutive of knowledge). Assuming that the *Zhuangzi* maintains a consistent position on the subject of emotions, then it is significant that *Zhuangzi* 5/55–60 does not advocate ceasing to emote.[12] Like this interpretation of the Mengsun passage, *Zhuangzi* 5/55–60 merely promotes not letting one's emotions cause oneself harm, which seems to amount to limiting, rather than eradicating, them. In sum, consistently reading *shi* as "authentic" can produce peculiar interpretations of passages, whereas consistently reading *shi* as fulfillment/fruit seems to avoid this problem.

As this discussion shows, the use of the character *shi* implies more of a sense of change and activity than translations like "reality" and "substance" tend to convey. Understood in terms of the notion of fruition, we see that the way *shi* functions implies a process of growth and increasing occupation of space. A container model stuffed with substances does not bring this activity to the fore. Terms that invoke illusion and nonexistence also fail to note the *process* involved in bringing something to fruition. In light of that process, the falseness that is sometimes associated with emptiness is the result of incomplete fruition. Something that is called *shi*, the *Mencius* reminds us, is brought to completion. On these grounds, it seems highly improbable that, in the Mengsun Cai passage, the term *shi* would refer to authenticity by virtue of an opposition to action (as if he "did the deed" but lacked the *shi*). With consistent interpretation of *shi* as fruition, activity seems central to the meaning of the term.

Ming/Shi as an Aural/Visual Pair

The distinctive role of *shi* 實 in sense discrimination is another factor that connects *shi* to change. Unlike reality, which may be accessible to all of the senses, *shi* is generally something seen by the eyes, in the same way that names are heard by the ears. In other words, in this section I argue that *ming/shi* is an aural/visual polarity. This point will be made by noting the various interconnections between the two pairs of terms—"speech and action" and "*ming* and *shi.*"

Whereas an empirical approach to 'reality' might define it in terms of access to the senses as a whole, *shi* is primarily accessible to sight. There is no indication that the senses collectively access *shi*. In fact, the five senses do not even seem to collectively verify knowledge.[13] The most common examples of testing knowledge in these texts involve tallying the ears' hearing with the eyes' seeing. Thus, most of the senses do not participate in verifying knowledge and most of the senses do not contact *shi*. The behavior of sense discrimination in these texts does not meet the expectation that reality is indicated by the character *shi*.

The emphasis on ears and eyes and their effects on the reception of the world (discussed in Chapter 2) should lend some initial credibility to the claim that *ming/shi* is an aural/visual pair. But before arguing that *shi* is visual in nature, the case must be made that *ming* is fundamentally aural/oral. What is controversial here is the texts' view of Chinese writing. My contention is that, within these early philosophical texts, *ming* 名 refers, first and foremost, to speech, and only incidentally to written characters as records of speech.

The use of sensory metaphors shows that *ming* 名 is consistently presented aurally/orally in Warring States philosophical texts. The texts contain no instances of *ming* being seen, while there are multiple instances of *ming* being heard and *ming* coming out of the mouth. In the most overt instance, the *Xunzi* 22/38 says that the function of a *ming* 名 is to be heard in such a way that makes *shi* understood.[14] Moreover, the substitution of *ming* 命 for *ming* 名 in *Mozi* 19/4–6 (see below) associates *ming* 名 with something inherently spoken (a decree).[15] Given the connection between these two *mings*, the *Mozi*'s argument against *ming* 命 implies that both terms refer to something that is not visible in nature. That is, *ming* 命 is so obviously not visible that the passage that argues against *ming* 命 cannot even use the phrase "seeing *ming*." Except when asserting that it is *not* possible to see *ming*, the *Mozi* resorts to strange phrases like "seeing the 'thing' (*wu* 物) of *ming*," and "seeing the 'body' (*ti* 體) of *ming*," in an attempt to find some aspect of *ming* that could possibly be visible:

> 然胡不嘗考之百姓之情
> 自古以及今生民以來者
> 亦嘗見命之物聞命之聲者乎
> 則未嘗有也
> 若以百姓為愚不肖耳目之情不足因而為法
> 然則胡不嘗考之諸候之傳言流語乎
> 自古以及今生民以來者
> 亦嘗有聞命之聲見命之體者乎則未嘗有也
>
> Then, why not try to test the *qing* [conditions? dispositions?] of the common people? From olden times

> until now, from the time that people have been born, has anyone ever *seen* the *wu* [thing] of *ming* [fate/ordainment/decree] or *heard* the sound of *ming*? Of course, no one has.
>
> If the common people are considered stupid and worthless, and the *qing* [conditions? dispositions?] of their ears and eyes are not reliable as a standard, then why not inquire into the recorded speech of the feudal lords that has flowed down to us? From olden times until now, from the time that people have been born, has any of them ever *heard* the sound of *ming* or *seen* the body [*ti*] of *ming*? Of course, none of them has.
>
> (*Mozi* 36/6–9)

Translating this passage's first visual reference to *ming* as "such a thing as *ming*" (or some other equally smooth locution) would obscure the pattern here. The parallelism in the passage requires some visual aspect of *ming* to correspond to the aurality of its sound. Not satisfied with its first attempt (*wu* of *ming*), the passage tries "*ti* of *ming*" the second time. The text's fumbling with "*wu* of *ming*" followed by "*ti* of *ming*" indicates that *wu* and *ti* are visual items (a point of relevance later in this argument). At the same time, it indicates that *ming* is not normally viewed as having a visual aspect. If it were, the text would have settled on it.

Evidence of various other sorts speaks in favor of the theory that names are oral/aural. One could read Canon A 78 of the reconstructed Neo-Mohist Canons as saying that all sounds emitted by the mouth "have a *ming*":

> **A 78** 名達類私
> （名）〔物〕達也有實必待*之（多）*名也
> 命之〔馬〕類也〔若實〕也者必以是名也
> 命之〔臧〕私也是名也止於是實也
> 聲出口俱有名（若姓（宇）*字）

> C. *Ming* (name). Unrestricted: classifying: private.
> E. 'Thing' is 'unrestricted'; any object necessarily requires this name. Naming something 'horse' is 'classifying'; for 'like the object' we necessarily use this name. Naming someone 'Jack' is 'private'; this name stays confined in this object. The sounds which issue from the mouth all have the name. (For example, surname and style-name.)[16]
> (Graham, *Later Mohist Logic, Ethics and Science*, 325)

Whatever this might mean, it does seem to assert that "name" can be applied to any sound coming from the mouth. The *Shuo wen jie zi* says something similar regarding the constitution of the character—explaining *ming* 名 by saying 從口從夕 (derived from "mouth" and from "dark").[17] The term *ming* 名 also seems related to the less semantic, but certainly oral, *ming* 鳴 (calling) in the *Zhuangzi*, that appears when "Confucius" offers the following obscure advice:

> 吾語若若能入遊其樊而無感其名
> 入則鳴不入則止
> I will tell you. You can enter and roam in his enclosure, but don't stimulate his naming. If you enter, then call [*ming* 鳴], if not then stop.[18]
> (*Zhuangzi* 4/29–30)

The passage implies some kind of echo-response connection between a birdlike "calling" and the use of names (*ming* 名). Both this passage and those above support the claim that names (*ming* 名) refer broadly to sounds that come out of the mouth.[19] Thus, *ming* seems to be aural in nature.

Having argued thus far that *ming* is aural, it remains to be argued that *shi* is visual. The visuality of *shi* appears in certain passages that substitute *ming* and *xing* (name and action) and *yan* and *shi* (speech and *shi*), instead of the usual *yan* and *xing* and *ming* and *shi*.[20] Some of these puzzling passages that pair speech and *shi* become more comprehensible when viewing *shi* as (a visible act of) fulfillment, rather than as reality.[21] More importantly, simply by implying a parallel relation between the two pairs—*yan/xing* and *ming/shi*—these passages lend credence to the idea that *ming/shi* is an aural/visual pair.

Just as one's speech may be enacted (*xing*), so too one's speech may be fulfilled (*shi*) through action. For example, the *Mencius* 4B17 constructs *yan* and *shi* into a pair, like *yan/xing* or *ming/shi*:

> 言無實不祥
> 不祥之實蔽賢者當之
> Speech without *shi* [fulfillment] is inauspicious, and beclouding the virtuous is equivalent to an inauspicious *shi*.[22]
> (*Mencius* 4B17)

The passage is less puzzling if we think of "speech" here as a promise (or perhaps a reputation, as in *ming*/name) and *shi* as actions (as in *xing*/act) that fulfill the reputation. We might interpret the first line as saying that speech not fulfilled by action is unlucky. The second line then supplies an act of fulfilling that is itself unlucky—the act of obscuring the virtuous. Such a reading has advantages over reading *shi* as "reality." "Beclouding the virtuous" seems more likely to be described as an act than as a reality. Moreover, if *shi* were "reality" or even "the facts," then the failure to match speech and *shi* should be called "inaccurate" rather than "inauspicious." The normative tenor of the example (the reference to obscuring the virtuous) also points to something other than a factual failure.

In another example of *yan* and *shi* (*Zhuangzi* 4/49–50), speech is paired with action, which is explicitly associated with *shi*. The *Zhuangzi* 4/49–50 says that speech is like wind and waves and implies that action (*xing* 行) either loses (*sang* 喪) it or "*shi*-es" 實 it.[23] In addition to implying that *shi* fulfills speech through action, the passage characterizes *shi* as the swelling of a wave—thus presenting *shi* as extending in space. The opposite of *shi* here is not unreality, but loss (perhaps the deflation of a retreating wave). Thus, like the case discussed above, this passage argues for interpreting *shi* on the model of *xing*—as action that fills out speech.[24]

Along with these connections of *yan* and *shi*, the uses of *shi* in the *Mozi* provide particularly good evidence for interpreting *shi* as visually accessible action.[25] The *Mozi* speaks generally of the *shi* of both the eyes and ears, but when it breaks down the compound, *ming* is what is heard and *shi* is what is seen.

Some of the *Mozi* evidence for the visuality of *shi* occurs in its analogies involving blind people. One such analogy makes use of this subtle aural/visual contrast:

> 今天下之諸候將猶多皆免攻伐並兼
> 則是有譽義之名而不察其實也
> 此譬猶盲者之與人同命白黑之名
> 而不能分其物也
> 則豈謂有別哉
>
> Now the world's feudal lords still attack and assault each other. This is to have praise for the name of righteousness, without investigating its *shi* [its fulfillment?]. This resembles the way a blind person, along with others, similarly ordains [*ming* 命] the names [*ming* 名] of black and white, but cannot discriminate their *wu* [the things that correspond to them?]. Can this be said to be having discrimination?
> (*Mozi* 19/4–6)

The passage shows that *wu* (thing) can substitute for *shi*. (It first mentions "investigating its *shi*," and then puts "discriminat[e] their *wu*" in its place.) As *Mozi* 36/7 indicates (see page 57), the *wu* here that cannot be discriminated is visual in nature.[26] Moreover, while comparison to *Mozi* 36/7 suggests that *wu* and *shi* are visual, the reference to ordaining suggests that *ming* is aural. In other words, the passage claims that a blind person can sense *ming* (the correlate of the aural sense); however, he/she cannot sense *shi* and/or *wu* (its visual counterpart). Finally, the passage implies some kind of visual analogy between righteous *shi* and black and white things. In both cases, the blind person, while able to utter their names, cannot see the differences.

Another blind–person analogy in *Mozi* 47/23 illustrates that "seeing the difference" depends on action. The passage compares the act of picking black and white (things) to the articulation of a name:

> 今瞽曰鉅者白也黔者墨也
> 雖明目者無以易之
> 兼白黑使瞽取焉不能知也
> 故我曰瞽不知白黑者非以其名也以其取也
> Now, the blind say that what is bright is white, and what is dark is black. Even the clear-sighted would not change that. But if you mix together white and black and cause blind people to pick [among them], they are not able to know [how to do it].[27] Therefore, when I say that the blind do not know white and black, it is not with regard to their use of names, it is with regard to their picking.
> (*Mozi* 47/23–24)

Although the passage does not mention either *shi* or *wu*, it clearly echoes *Mozi* 19/4–6. Here, instead of "investigation of *shi*" and "discrimination of *wu*," we have picking out black from white. On the grounds of the similarity between this passage and 19/4–6, we might expect that here too there is an implicit *shi* that matches the names black and white. We might initially suppose that the unstated *shi* in this passage are black and white things. But a closer reading argues for a different conclusion. First, black and white stand on their own. In contrast to what might be expected in a substance-based metaphysics, no word for "thing/object" even appears. Second, in the last line, the comparison is not between names and things, but between names and picking.[28] Like 19/4–6, which identifies an act of righteousness as a visual counterpart for the name of righteousness, this too identifies a visual act: the act of picking. Whereas speech is the aural evidence that a person can use names, the act of picking is the visual evidence. Once again, in a substance-based metaphysics, the significant visual element would be the objects, which possess properties of being black and white. But here the act of picking (which is the proof of eyesight) counts more. The use of a blind person in both of these passages manages to highlight both the visuality of *shi* and its connection to action.

In addition to highlighting the visuality of *shi*, the *Mozi* also contains passages suggesting an aural/visual aspect to the *ming/shi* pair. In the *Mozi*, examples of aural/visual patterns that use *wu* rather than *shi* are more common. One example that parallels *ming* and *wu* concerns the sound and the *wu* (visual aspect?) of ghosts and spirits. The *Mozi* asks,

> ...生民以來者亦有嘗見鬼神之物聞鬼神之聲則鬼神何謂無乎
> [If]...since the beginning of humanity, there are also those who have seen the *wu* of ghosts and spirits, and heard the voices of ghosts and spirits, how can they be called "absent"?
> (*Mozi* 31/12–13)

Here, instead of "the sound and *wu* of *ming*" (*Mozi* 36/6 above), we have "the sound and *wu* of ghosts and spirits." (Again, translating this as "*such things as* ghosts and spirits" would obscure the aural/visual pattern in these examples.) The use of these different pairs—sound and *wu* (*Mozi* 31/12, 36/6), sound and *ti* (*Mozi* 36/9), *ming* and *wu* (19/5), and *ming* and *shi* (19/5)—in each case, more or less obviously in the context of things heard and seen, implies that *shi*, like other pairs for *ming* and sound, is something visible. Therefore, in the *Mozi*, *ming* and *shi* seem to fit the pattern of aural and visual parallel pairings, like *yan* and *xing*. *Ming* is something sensed by the ears, and so too *shi* seems to be something sensed by the eyes.

Indeed, *ming* and *shi* resemble *yan* and *xing* in one other significant way—their union seems to contribute to knowledge. As noted in Chapters 2 and 3, the philosophical texts of the period tend to presume that speech and action should match like two parts of a tally. The *Mozi*'s version of this refers to their matching by using the term *he* 合 (uniting) (*Mozi* 16/29). Similarly, the *Mozi* describes the ideal relation of *ming* and *shi* using the term "uniting." According to the *Mozi*, *ming* and *shi* unite by "mating":

> 所以謂名也所謂實也名實耦合也
> That by which something is called is the name. What is called is the *shi*. The mating of name and *shi* is uniting.[29] (*Mozi* 42/37)

Thus, the same term that depicts the relation of speech to action also depicts the relation of names to *shi*. As noted in Chapter 3, like speech and action, names and *shi* are invoked in the context of standards of measure. Because standards of measure facilitate reliable knowing, it may be significant that this line from the *Mozi* appears to belong to a passage concerning knowledge.[30] On these grounds, it could be argued that standardized matching of *ming* and *shi* produces knowledge, following the same pattern that produces knowledge by reliably matching speech and action.

Hence, a variety of evidence contributes to the proposition that *ming/shi* is an aural/visual pair: Consistent references to hearing and speaking *ming* imply that *ming* is (at least fundamentally, if not exclusively) something spoken and heard. At the same time, parallels between *ming* and *shi* imply that *shi* is primarily visual in nature. In addition, some troublesome passages containing the character *shi* seem more coherent when *shi* is interpreted in terms of (visible) acts of fulfillment. The import of these factors, which argue for interpreting *ming/shi* as an aural/visual pair, is enhanced by the possibility that uniting *ming* and *shi* produces knowledge. In sum, rather than view *shi* as reality, a better understanding of the texts might result from viewing it as the active, visual counterpart to hearing sounds.

Ming/Shi and the Rectification of Names

The discussion of the "rectification of names" (*zhengming* 正名) in the *Lunyu* 13/3 and in *Xunzi* 22 can be used in favor of the argument that *ming/shi* is an aural/visual pair. The view that *ming/shi* should be understood as names/reality is in tension with the notion of rectification of names. If reality is truly real, and names are not part of it, then correcting names is not likely to have much of an effect on it. This problem might be resolved by arguing that names do not *describe* a preexistent reality, but rather *prescribe* what reality is to be like.[31] But to the extent that this means reality is determined by something external to it, the term "reality" itself seems dubious. In the discussion of rectifying names, it seems even more important than usual to get our own terminology right. If names create reality, then names might be more real than what they create. At the very least, it seems that names are equally as real as what they create. With this question about ontological status-equivalence in mind, this section explores how the texts present interactions between names and *shi*. It argues that the relation between names and *shi* is two-sided, with no inherently superior side. And yet, when it comes to restoring order, it is names that are subject to correction. Working from aural/visual parallels and metaphors related to names and *shi*, the section proposes a justification for the importance placed on correcting names.

The *Lunyu* and the *Xunzi* seem far more interested in correcting names than they are in correcting the counterpart of names (however conceived).[32] The *Xunzi* contains an entire chapter devoted to the topic of correcting names, asserting that correct names instituted by true rulers will bring about proper governing. For its part, the *Lunyu*'s attention to the topic makes up in enthusiasm what it lacks in quantity. The rectification of names passage in the *Lunyu* invests enormous confidence in the efficacy of correcting names. When asked about his first priority for administering a state, Confucius is reported to have replied,

> 必也正名乎....
> 名不正則言不順言不順則事不成
> 事不成則禮樂不興
> 禮樂不興則刑罰不中
> 刑罰不中則民無所錯手足
> 故君子名之必可言也言之必可行也
> 君子於其言無所苟而已矣
> Certainly, correct the names....
> If names are not correct, then speech is not smooth. If speech is not smooth, then events are not completed. If events are not completed, then ritual and music do not flourish. If ritual and music do not flourish, then laws and punishments are not on target. If laws and punishments are not on target, then the people have nowhere to place hand and foot. Therefore, noble people's naming must be speakable, their speech must be enactable. With regard to speech, the noble person is in no way careless.
> (*Lunyu* 13/3)

Of course, there are multiple cases in all the texts wherein *ming* and *shi* are weighed against one another, but this notion of "rectifying names" stands out. It seems a bit inexplicable that the *Lunyu* and the *Xunzi* adopt this program expressly aimed at naming.

In order to understand the conception of names, we might look at the metaphors relating names and *shi*. Rather than saying that names "picture" or "mirror" things (which implies a reproductive, secondary status), the texts tend to use terms that cluster around the metaphor of "binding" to describe the relation between names and *shi*. The *Xunzi* describes a disruptive relation of names and *shi* as being "knotted" (22/13).[33] Ideally, this knotty relation is a straightforward bond. But it is significant that both sides are subject to being bound. In some cases, the relation of names and *shi* seems as if the *shi* were there first. The *Zhengming* provides an example of this:

> 故知者為之分別制名以指實
> 上以明貴賤
> 下以辨同異
> 貴賤明同異別
> Therefore those who are knowledgeable for this reason divide and separate and establish names in order to point to *shi*.
> Above, to clarify noble and base, below, to distinguish same and different.
> (*Xunzi* 22/14–15)

Here, names have an ostensive relation to *shi*—"pointing" to *shi* that are noble, base, similar, or different—as if names were bound to *shi*. But the *Zhengming* also mentions a type of binding wherein *shi* are bound by names:

> 名也者所以期累實也
> As for names, they are that which meet and bind *shi*.[34]
> (*Xunzi* 22/38–39)

Perhaps examples of names binding *shi* might include cases where deeds are turned to the benefit of reputation. For instance, a fictitious Confucius in the *Zhuangzi* notes that desire for fame fosters remarkable acts of bravery:

> 夫保始之徵不懼之實勇士一人雄入於九軍
> 將求名而能自要者而猶若是
> 而況...心未嘗死者乎

> The test of protecting the beginning [or "what one starts with"] is *shi* [acting/fulfilling a name] without being afraid: a single brave knight boldly entering a battle of the nine armies. If someone seeking a name can demand this of himself, and be like this, how much more so...one whose heartmind never dies?!
> (*Zhuangzi* 5/11–13)

With something akin to begrudging admiration, the passage shows how deeds can be performed in the service of a name (which, thus, antedates the deed).[35] The *Zhengming* describes yet another option—an interrelated process in which *shi* are bound by names, and, in virtue of this, names are bound by *shi*:

> 名無固實約之以命實
> 約定俗成謂之實名
> 名有固善徑易而不拂謂之善名
> Names have no original *shi* [filling?]. Bind them by ordaining *shi*.[36] If the binding settles and a habit forms, call it a *shi* name [a full name? a productive name?].
> Names do have original goodness. If it is direct, easy, and not contrary, call it a good name.[37]
> *Xunzi* 22/26–27

Looking carefully at the second and third lines, *as the shi are named*, the names themselves become bound to the *shi* (which is why they become "*shi* names"). It is as if the binding of the *shi* (naming them) is concomitant with binding the names. Thus, both names and *shi* are in some sense "bound" in these attachments. We may see this as evidence that it is not the case that names merely reflect or re-present *shi*. Thus far, it seems that names and *shi* occupy equal footing.

Arguments to the contrary often point to the supposed parasitic aspect of names in one particular passage from the *Zhuangzi*. The *Zhuangzi* reports the comments of a person who refuses to occupy an office for the sake of a name that is already fulfilled. He says,

> 子治天下天下既已治也
> 而我猶代子吾將為名乎
> 名者實之賓也吾將為賓乎
> You're ordering the world, and the world is already ordered; if I were to take your place, would it be for the sake of the name? The name is the guest of the *shi*. Would it be for the sake of the guest?
> (*Zhuangzi* 1/24–25)

The speaker compares the relation of *shi* and name to that of host and guest. However, it would be wrong to read this as affirming the superiority of *shi*. The first line points to a *shi* that is already filled—the position of ordering the world. Because that position is filled, the only position available is that of the guest. Although a host may seem more important than a guest, the passage identifies names as *honored* visitors (using the polite term *bin* 賓). Thus, the name visits the *shi*, like a guest of honor, in a relation of mutual respect.[38] The recluse refuses the position of guest, not because it is inferior, but because it is the only position available to refuse.

In fact, respectful relations of host to guest are typical of the formalized, even ritualized, relations between *shi* and names. As in the context of ritual, repeated patterns of use produce order in the mutual bonds between names and *shi*—that is, the original situation (wherein *shi* are named) is stabilized by a gradual process of habitual attachment. This ceremonial attachment connotes decorum and ethical correctness. The *Xunzi*'s preceding reference to "appropriateness" (*yi* 宜) in naming (*Xunzi* 22/25) hints at questions of ethical and ceremonial decorum. In fact, "binding" is the term that the ethically ideal Yan Hui purportedly uses to describe the effects of Confucius's ritual teaching:

> 博我以文約我以禮
> He broadened me with culture and bound me with ritual.
> (*Lunyu* 9/11)

Perhaps just as ritual gradually binds Yan Hui to upright behaviors, so too the habitual use of names gradually binds an ethically correct order to their relation to certain *shi*. Like guests and hosts, names and *shi* are bound by a ritual context that would counteract any tendencies to stray off into unpredictability. In other words, the attachment of names and *shi* may belong to the context of an organized and ritualized process of ethical enhancement. (Hence the term for "correcting" names is also used to connote ethical correctness.) The ritualized setting highlights that the connection between names and *shi* is orderly and reliable (and by no means parasitic).

The metaphor of guest and host not only sets names and *shi* in a ritualized context, it also indicates the particular feature of names that accounts for why they elicit correcting. Like a guest, names seem to be less "grounded" than *shi*, and more inclined to move. On the same lines, the fact that names are said to be "added to" or "located in" *shi*, conveys an impression that a name takes up less space, so to speak.[39] As the *Mozi* mentions, individual names seem to stop or stay within the confines of certain *shi*:

> 是名也止於是實也
> This name stays in this *shi*.
> (*Mozi* 42/35)

The implication of this stopping is that names have more potential than *shi* to move on. The implication is similar when the *Xunzi* mentions names, rather than *shi*, as being "settled."[40] As *Xunzi* 22/26 (see above) makes clear—names have the capacity to be *shi*-like (to be *shi* names), whereas the same is not said of *shi*, that is, *shi* are not described as name-like (named *shi*?). Thus, names are more flexible in relation to *shi* than vice versa. Names have the potential to be either full or empty, and it is easy for something flexible (or tenuous) to travel.

In contrast to the flexible emptiness of names, the metaphor inherent in the notion of *shi* as fruit evokes a certain gradual slowness. The *Lunyu* stipulates that fruits occur only gradually—not arriving until after flowers, if they arrive at all:[41]

> 苗而不秀者有矣夫秀而不實者有矣夫
> There are indeed seedlings that do not flower, and there are flowers that do not fruit.
> (*Lunyu* 9/22)

In addition to coming slowly, fruit has a characteristic heaviness that can only impede its speed. The *Laozi* implies that *shi* is also relatively "thick" in character. The passage aligns *shi* with the thickness of fruit, in contrast to the thinness of flowers:[42]

> 是以大丈夫居其厚而不居其泊
> 居其實不居其華
> Therefore, the great man dwells in the thick and does not dwell in the thin; dwells in the fruit and does not dwell in the flower.
> (*Laozi* 38)

A passage from the *Yuan Dao* chapter of the *Huainanzi* (dating from the early Han and therefore questionable as evidence here) hints at the relative "heaviness" of earthbound *shi* by contrasting it with birds flying in the air:

> 鳥排虛而飛獸蹠實而走
> Birds fly by stroking emptiness.
> Animals run by treading *shi*.[43]

Although names are not always empty, their flexible potential to move contrasts sharply with the slowness and heaviness of *shi*.

While heaviness of *shi* is associated with the earth, names have more affinity with the air. They benefit from being carried on the wind, which, the *Xunzi* notes, amplifies sound:

> 順風而呼聲非加疾也
> 而聞者彰
> When you accord with the wind and shout, the sound is no stronger, and yet the audibility is amplified.
> (*Xunzi* 1/7)

As argued in Chapter 2, the wind is a force of disruption, with a potency that notably affects those who contact it. But names also hang in the air in a positive sense—as scalelike standards of measure. The *Xunzi* says,

> 名聲未足以縣天下
> [Their] name and sound is not sufficient to hang over the world [as a balancing force].[44]
> (*Xunzi* 9/99)

While names may not exactly fly, they do move "at the speed of sound" so to speak. The *Lunyu* bemoans this capacity in reference to speech:

> 子貢曰惜乎夫子之說君子也駟不及舌
> Zigong commented, "It is a pity that the gentleman should have spoken so about the gentleman. 'A team of horses cannot catch up with one's tongue.'"
> (*Lunyu* 12/8)

In addition to speed, names also partake in the peculiar responsiveness of sound.[45] In sum, names contrast to *shi* like the heavens above to the earth below, or the tenuous to the filled out. Names have the greater speed and flexibility. To that extent, it is both more important to counter their influence, and more feasible to alter their state.

Conclusions

I have argued that *ming* and *shi* are an aural and visual pair. As such, their relations are parallel to one another, and their importance seems equivalent. Yet names are the focus of rectification, for reasons that might relate to the aurality of names. In contrast to action, which moves with the heaviness of earth, names occupy little space and travel lightly. The reason why rulers must take unauthorized names particularly seriously is that names travel with the speed of sound, like speech, which is inclined to bypass action, because of its greater speed and fluidity. As a result, speech must slow down if it is to match action like two parts of a tally. So too names must slow down, perhaps so that names and *shi* may function as foundations for knowledge and proper standards for measure.

Chapter 5: Conclusion

As a measure of the usefulness of this project, this Conclusion aims to employ this study of the senses to illuminate some underlying differences in the arguments of certain Warring States texts. In particular, this Conclusion will illustrate points where the *Xunzi* contrasts with the *Mencius* and the *Laozi* contrasts with the *Zhuangzi*. In the first section, I will show, by means of an analysis of their treatment of hearing and seeing, that the *Xunzi* and the *Mencius* ground knowledge differently. In the second section, by exploring their unusual approaches to the senses, I will sort out how the *Laozi* and the *Zhuangzi* reach different positions about their use.

Hopefully, the overall project will gain some justification insofar as its analysis of the senses can elucidate the contrasts considered in this Conclusion. In other words, this Conclusion may serve as a test of the accuracy of my analysis of sense discrimination in these texts.

Comparison of the *Xunzi* and the *Mencius*

While aural/visual parallels occur in all of the Warring States philosophical texts, in the *Xunzi* they play an especially prominent role. For the *Xunzi* the responses of the eyes and ears produce reliable knowledge, both because they correspond to one another, and because they respond spontaneously to stimulation. While spontaneity of this sort precludes the labor of selecting an appropriate response, it does not preclude evaluating responses in relation to their consequences. This indeed reflects the *Xunzi*'s pragmatic approach to knowledge. In the *Xunzi*, knowledge is oriented toward embodiment and action. By contrast, in the *Mencius*, origin plays a greater role than consequences. When the *Mencius* treats aural and visual parallels, it shows greater interest in how these senses are rooted in the heartmind. Likewise, spontaneity of the senses is quite a different matter in the *Mencius*. For the *Mencius*, spontaneity has to do with reflecting the heartmind. It is less a response than an extension. Thus, the *Xunzi* and the *Mencius* attribute the reliability of aural/visual pairs to different causes—for the *Xunzi*, spontaneous response; for the *Mencius*, spontaneous extension of the heartmind.

The Xunzi

The *Xunzi* treats the eyes and ears as things that respond and correspond. The *Xunzi*'s aural and visual pairs often consist of echoes and shadows. In the *Xunzi*'s usage, these metaphors tend to emphasize spontaneity of response. That is, the *Xunzi* does not employ them to indicate dubious ontological status. Instead, the *Xunzi* emphasizes the automatic nature of the responses of echoes and shadows. For example, the *Xunzi* compares the ruler's moral responses to echoes and shadows. Although it notes that people in superior roles teach those who are below, it does not imply that the response of those below is somehow illusory or false. In fact, the shadow/echo response is appropriate precisely because all it does is respond:

> 上者下之師也夫下之和上
> 譬之猶響之應聲影之像形也...
> Those above are the teachers of those below. The way those below harmonize with those above is like, for example, the way an echo responds to a sound and the shadow has the shape of a form...
> (*Xunzi* 16/77–78)

The *Xunzi* dwells on speed and spontaneity when it describes a good government as one in which the people imitate and respond to the ruler like shadows and echoes:

> 政令教化形下如影應卒遇變齊給如響
> Their government orders and instructions for transformation are modeled below like a shadow. They respond promptly to sudden change with quick speed, like an echo.[1]
> (*Xunzi* 13/5)

The *Xunzi* also compares the common people's responses to the ruler with the responses involved in singing (auditory) and in using a gnomon (visual). The people respond spontaneously, as long as the form is displayed.[2]

> 主者民之唱也上者下之儀也
> 彼將聽唱而應視儀而動
> 唱默則民無應也
> 儀隱則下無動也
> 不應不動則上下無以相有也
> The ruler is the people's singing master. Those above are the model instrument for those below. They listen to the singing master, then respond. They look at the instrument, then move. If the singing master is silent, then the people have nothing to respond to. If the model is dark, then those below have nothing to move with. If there's no response and no movement, then it's like above and below having no relations at all.
> (*Xunzi* 18/1–2)

In sum, aurality and visuality in the *Xunzi* indicate spontaneous responsiveness.

In fact, correspondence and response are fundamental to the *Xunzi*'s view of knowledge. The *Xunzi* describes knowledge in terms of responses:

知通乎大道應變而不窮
辨乎萬物之情性者也
The knowledge [of worthies] communes with the great way, responds and changes and does not reach a limit, and divides the *qingxing* [dispositional nature?] of the ten thousand things.
(*Xunzi* 31/17)

The metaphor for the 'correspondence' (*dang* 當) of knowing seems to be a road to which knowledge responds.[3]

以義變應知當曲直故也
[The gentleman] changes and responds through righteousness, because his knowledge corresponds to the crooked and straight.
(*Xunzi* 3/15)

Hence, for the *Xunzi*, knowledge itself amounts to corresponding responses.

As in the examples of echoes and shadows, a knowledgeable response in the *Xunzi* seems to be one that occurs spontaneously. The *Xunzi* stresses that responses should be timely. It notes that one should respond as things "arrive" (happen):

當時則動物至而應
事起而辨治亂可否
昭然明矣
When the time corresponds, then act; when things arrive, respond; when events occur, then discriminate. Order and disorder, proper and improper, will become patently clear.
(*Xunzi* 21/93)

The *Xunzi* states explicitly that the proper response does *not* involve forethought. Appropriate responses simply happen, in a timely and smooth manner.[4] Moreover, the *Xunzi* suggests that the responses that meet the changes of time happen easily, like counting one and two:

> 脩百王之法若辨黑白
> 應當時之變若數一二...
> when one cultivates the model of the Hundred Kings like distinguishing black from white, and when one responds appropriately to every change of circumstances like counting one, two...
> (*Xunzi* 8/59–60)

Perhaps because it is easy, the response does not wear itself out.[5] In other words, knowledge may be derived from spontaneous responses because they are simple and unforced.

In keeping with this sense of spontaneity, the reliability of the eyes and ears does not even depend upon looking and listening. In one case, the *Xunzi* says the eyes and ears of the gentleman can dispense entirely with the effort of looking and listening:

> 不視而見不聽而聰不言而信不慮而知
> 不動而功告至備也
> 天子也者埶至重形至佚心至愈
> He does not look yet sees; does not listen yet hears; does not speak yet is trusted; does not ponder yet knows; does not move yet achieves. His announcements are completely perfect. One who is a Son of Heaven: his strength is completely respected; his form is completely comfortable; his heartmind is completely at ease.
> (*Xunzi* 24/2–3)

It seems that looking and listening are not necessary, because the mutual resonance occurs spontaneously.[6] This may explain the *Xunzi*'s attitude toward the unseen and unheard. Instead of advocating investigation of the unseen and unheard in order to respond properly to them, the *Xunzi* warns the rulers and ministers against overtaxing the senses (see *Xunzi* 11/111–112, page 42). Specifically, the *Xunzi* is opposed to the effort of *extending* knowledge, speech, and action:

> 知不務多務審其所知
> 言不務多務審其所謂
> 行不務多務審其所由
> Knowledge should not strive for more, but strive to examine what it knows. Speech should not strive for more, but strive to examine what is spoken of. Action should not strive for more, but strive to examine from whence it comes.
> (*Xunzi* 31/10–11)

According to the *Xunzi*, some things (such as "the mutual operations and alternations of fullness and emptiness, the separations and distinctions of hard and white and same and different," 若夫充虛之相施易也堅白同異之分隔也, *Xunzi* 8/34) simply exceed the boundaries of the sage's knowledge. These alternations and distinctions that are beyond the limits of knowledge are beyond the limits of the ear and eye:

> 聰耳之所不能聽也
> 明目之所不能見也
> 辯士之所不能言也
> 雖有聖人之知未能僂指也
> [These are what] the keen ear cannot hear, the bright eye cannot see, and the well-spoken scholar cannot speak. Even if he possesses the knowledge of a sage, still he will be unable to "bend a finger" at them.[7]
> (*Xunzi* 8/34)

The *Xunzi* criticizes a ruler who tries to do small things by himself for transgressing the limits of the eyes and ears.[8] (See *Xunzi*

12/116–117, page 42.) This kind of criticism might simply mean that better discriminations result from mastery of a limited quantity.[9] But viewed in terms of the *Xunzi*'s emphasis on responsiveness, it is probable that, in the *Xunzi*, even subtle mastery of the discriminations at hand should be spontaneous and unforced. What seems noteworthy is that the *Xunzi* expects seeing, hearing, and knowing to be spontaneous and forbids transgressing the proper limits of these functions. In other words, the *Xunzi*'s strictures against extending sensory investigation also fit its model of spontaneous sensory response.

The *Xunzi*'s focus on spontaneous sensory responses is compatible with its pragmatic concerns. In the *Xunzi*, the alternative to reliable sight and hearing is not inaccurate sight and hearing, but danger and confusion. The *Xunzi* contrasts blindness to clarity of sight, deafness to keenness of hearing, ending the sequence with the contrast of danger and safety.

> 以盲為明以聾為聰以危為安
> He considers blindness as clarity, deafness as keenness, and danger as safety.
> (*Xunzi* 26/35)

Distinguishing colors with blind eyes or sounds with deaf ears produces confusion and chaos:

> 不是師法而好自用
> 譬之是猶以盲辨色
> 以聾辨聲也
> 舍亂妄無為也
> Not to take this as one's teacher and model, but instead favor one's own usage, is like using the blind to distinguish color, using the deaf to distinguish sounds. Apart from [causing] chaos and recklessness, it does nothing.
> (*Xunzi* 2/39–40)

Thus, the alternative to keenness and clarity is confusion, which amounts to danger. In other words, failure of the two senses that produce knowledge is assessed in terms of pragmatic considerations, rather than considerations of accuracy.

Judging hearing and seeing in terms of their consequences is an extension of the idea that knowing itself is not the final aim. The *Xunzi* states that knowing is superior to hearing and seeing, but not as good as acting, whereas acting is better than knowing, seeing, *and* hearing:[10]

> 不聞不若聞之
> 聞之不若見之
> 見之不若知之
> 知之不若行之
> 學至於行之而後止矣
> Not hearing is not as good as hearing something, hearing it is not as good as seeing it, seeing it is not as good as knowing it, knowing it is not as good as enacting it. Study goes as far as enacting it, and then it stops.[11]
> (*Xunzi* 8/102–103)

This ranking suggests something in the distance gradually becoming more internalized. That is, the only difference between seeing and hearing that the *Xunzi* explicitly notes is that the eye's range is closer than that of the ear.[12] Thus, viewing the ranking in this light, hearing, seeing, knowing, and enacting might indicate things becoming increasing near and finally being enacted in oneself.

This movement from the distant to the near may be elucidated by another passage that is also related to study. In this passage, the progression is directed toward beautifying or embellishing the body/person:[13]

> 君子之學也入乎耳箸乎心
> 布乎四體形乎動靜
> 端而言蝡而動一可以為法則

小人之學也入乎耳出乎口
口耳之間則四寸耳
曷足以美七尺之軀

The gentleman's study enters through the ear, is apparent in the heartmind, is located in the four limbs, and is shaped in his movement and rest. In the slightest speech and smallest movement, it can be taken as model and rule. The small person's study enters in the ear and exits from the mouth. The space between the ear and the mouth is a mere four inches. How can this be sufficient to embellish seven feet of body?
(*Xunzi* 1/30–32)

Here, what the gentleman hears becomes manifest in aural and visual responses that mark a transformation of the entire body/person. This embellishment of the person seems to have something to do with knowing. In another passage, right after "collectively knowing the ten thousand things" and before the "singular identification of a kind" (which seem to be two poles of the knowing process), the *Xunzi* mentions that the body/person will be adorned or beautified:

以贊稽之萬物可兼知也
身盡其故則美
類不可兩也
故知者擇一而壹焉

By considering comparatively, the ten thousand things can be collectively known. When the body/person exhausts its *gu*, it is embellished. "Of a kind" cannot be two. Therefore the knower selects one and has oneness.[14]
(*Xunzi* 21/49–50)

These bodily embellishment passages help explain how the *Xunzi* ranks knowing. It values knowing not in itself, but for the changes it can affect. The progression in the passage that ranks hearing, seeing, knowing, and acting does not simply reaffirm that hearing and seeing function in the service of knowing. It suggests that hearing, seeing, *and* knowing all work in the service of embodying.[15] Thus, embodying the way and allowing it to transform oneself is the goal of knowing. The *Xunzi* says,

> 知道察知道行體道者也
> One who knows the way of examining, and knows the way of acting, embodies the way.
> (*Xunzi* 21/40)

Thus, in the *Xunzi*, knowledge itself works in the service of transformative embodiment.

The *Xunzi* depicts knowledge as a kind of response and emphasizes corresponding aural and visual responses. Its stress on the spontaneity of these responses leaves little room for strenuous calculated analysis. In fact, the *Xunzi* endorses timely responses and explicitly rejects strained effort in the areas of looking and listening. The *Xunzi* implies that hearing, seeing, and knowing should be evaluated on the basis of their results—a consequentially focused perspective that coincides with the *Xunzi*'s view of knowing as embodied transformation. Thus, we can see in the *Xunzi* the Warring States texts' shared view of the senses working to support the *Xunzi*'s specific evaluative criteria for knowledge.

The Mencius

The *Mencius*'s criteria for evaluating reliable speech and action is quite different from the *Xunzi's*. In certain passages, the *Mencius* states that action need not produce consequences and speech need not rectify action or even be trustworthy. These striking differences between the *Mencius* and the *Xunzi* can be explained by the *Mencius*'s approach to the senses. Although it focuses on the aural and visual senses, the *Mencius* does not describe them in terms of responses. Instead, the *Mencius* emphasizes that what we hear and see in people originates in their heartminds. Hence, it describes aural and visual aspects of a person in terms of how they reflect their origins. Both texts emphasize spontaneity, but in the two texts spontaneous movement flows in different directions. The *Xunzi*'s spontaneity does not originate in any particular place. By contrast, the *Mencius* emphasizes the heartmind, which spontaneously extends to the body's periphery and beyond. This is evident in another area of contrast between the *Mencius* and the *Xunzi*. Whereas the *Xunzi* devotes an entire chapter to discrediting the practice of reading physiognomy, the *Mencius* seems sympathetic to physiognomic principles. That is, the *Mencius* trusts that the visible and auditory aspects of a person will reflect their common origin.

The *Mencius* asserts that a great person's speech does not have to be trustworthy and a great person's actions do not have to produce results:[16]

> 大人者言不必信行不必果惟義所在
> In the great person, speech need not be trustworthy, actions need not be productive.[17] They must only be located in what is right.
> (*Mencius* 4B11)

In a description of the proper attitude for mourning, the *Mencius* also states that speech should not aim to rectify action:

> 經德不回非以干祿也言語必信非以正行也
> 君子行法以俟命而已矣
> Go straight in virtue without turning, not in order to seek emolument. Speech and words must be trustworthy, not in order to rectify action. The action and model of the

superior person awaits *ming* [fate/ordainment/decree] and that is all.
(*Mencius* 7B33)

The notion that actions need not be productive seems congruent with the claim that speech need not be aimed at rectifying action. There is some confusion regarding trustworthiness, however, because, unlike Mencius 4B11, this description of a great person insists that speech must be trustworthy. But despite the confusion about trustworthiness, the general force of these passages seems to be that attention to consequences is not necessary.

What seems to be more important in the *Mencius* is that, at least in some cases, speech and action should not be measured by their consequences. The *Mencius* seems to argue that there should be some *other* basis for evaluating speech and action. It offers two criteria for evaluating speech. The first is that it be concerned with the concise:

博學而詳說之將以反說約也
Learn broadly and discuss/explain it in detail, in order to return to discussing/explaining the concise [the restricted].[18]
(*Mencius* 4B15)

The second criterion for evaluating speech is that it proceeds from near to far. With its basis in one's own body/self, it only subsequently influences the rest of the world:

言近而指遠者善言也
守約而施博者善道也
君子之言也不下帶而道存焉
君子之守修其身而天下平
Speech about the near that points to the far is skillful speech. Holding the basics and giving broadly is a skillful way. The speech of the superior person does not go below

> the belt, but the way is preserved within it. What the superior person holds on to is the cultivation of the body/self and thereby the whole world is tranquil.[19]
> (*Mencius* 7B32)

These cases show that the *Mencius* favors returning to conciseness and proceeding from the near. What these two directions might have in common is that they indicate the origin—rather than the outcome. This suggests that the *Mencius*'s supplementary criterion for evaluating speech is preserving its origin/base.

The *Mencius* emphasizes that the origin of both visual and audible expression is the heartmind. In contrast to *Xunzi* 1/30—where study comes into the ears, and makes it way through the heartmind and limbs, with no particular stress on the heartmind—the *Mencius* states explicitly that visual expression comes from the heartmind. For instance, things that are rooted in the gentleman's heartmind are manifest in his whole body:

> 君子所性仁義禮智
> 根於心其生色也睟然見於面
> 盎於背施於四體
> That which the gentleman takes as his nature is humaneness, righteousness, ritual, and wisdom. These are rooted in the heartmind and born in the complexion. They are manifest agreeably in the face, as forcefulness of the back, and they show themselves in the four limbs.
> (*Mencius* 7A21)

Moreover, as described in Chapter 3, the *Mencius* specifically refers to illicit speech as emerging from the heartmind. In addition, it seems that good speech is born in the heartmind, according to the *Mencius*. Mencius does not include any orthodox phrases in his defense of his claim to "know speech," but we can infer that he has some mastery of these as well. In the dialogue with King Xuan of

Qi, the king complains that upon considering his own action, he himself failed to "obtain" his own heartmind. He praises Mencius, however, whom he describes as personifying the expression about being able to gauge another person's heartmind. Elaborating on this point, the king explicitly ascribes Mencius's success (in attaining his heartmind) to using *speech* that draws upon the connections to his heartmind:

> 詩云他人有心予忖度之夫子之謂也
> 夫我乃行之反而求之不得吾心
> 夫子言之於我心有戚戚焉
> The *Book of Poetry* says, "It is the heartmind of the other person, but I gauge and measure it." This describes you, Master. I indeed did the thing, but when I returned my thoughts to seek it, I could not obtain my heartmind. When you, Master, *spoke* it, in my mind there was much consonance.
> (*Mencius* 1A7)

Thus, good and bad speech is connected to the heartmind, where it seems to be "born" or "instigated." Perhaps this explains the *Mencius*'s criteria for judging speech and action. Visual and auditory manifestations may be measured against something other than each other or their consequences—they may be measured against their correspondence to their origins in the heartmind.

Indeed, the *Mencius*'s treatment of sensory spontaneity suggests as much. The term for response (*ying* 應)—ubiquitous in the *Xunzi*—is barely evident in the *Mencius*.[20] Nonetheless, the *Mencius* does value spontaneity. Instead of responsiveness, a different spontaneous aspect of aurality and vision is evident in the *Mencius*. That is, the *Mencius* describes spontaneous extending—from the heartmind in the center to the borders of the body/person.[21] For example, the *Mencius* is critical of petty advisors whose expressions automatically manifest their feelings of disappointment:

> 予豈若是小丈夫然哉
> 諫於其君而不受則怒
> 悻悻然見於其面
> Am I like one of these little people? They admonish their ruler, and when the ruler does not accept their advice, they become angry, showing their grievances all over their faces.
> (*Mencius* 2B12)

But while it is critical of this facial display, the *Mencius* is confident that the face *does* in fact express what the heartmind is feeling. Upon seeing their parents' bodies eaten by foxes and wild cats, it says the ancients reacted in this way:

> 其顙有泚睨而不視夫泚也
> 非為人泚中心達於面目
> Their foreheads began to perspire, and they looked askance, unable to look. This perspiration was not due to others. It extended from the center of their heartminds to their faces and eyes.
> (*Mencius* 3A5)

With its origin in the heartmind, the progression of the embodied feeling reaches out to the extremities of the person. Thus, when the hands and feet are set in motion, this motion is born of emotions, which originate in the heartmind. Speaking of the *shi* 實 "fruits" of benevolence, righteousness, knowledge, ritual, and music, the *Mencius* says,

> 樂則生矣生
> 則惡可已也
> 惡可已則不知足之蹈之手之舞之

> Joy is then born, and when it is born, it is not possible to stop it. Because it can't be stopped, then, unknowingly, the feet tap and the arms wave.
> (*Mencius* 4A27)

The *Mencius* is confident that what one sees and hears in people springs inexorably from the condition of their heartminds in their center.

In light of this spontaneous movement, the *Mencius* suggests that one can expect a certain consistency between the heartmind and various other personal features. The *Mencius* is generally sympathetic with a notion that supports viewing physiognomy as a sign of character.[22] The connection between the heartmind's roots and its many branches is particularly evident in relation to things that are seen and heard. The *Mencius* implies that a king should look like a king:

> 孟子見梁襄王出語人曰望之不似人君就之而不見所畏焉
> Mencius went to see King Xiang of Liang. As he came out, he said to someone, "Looking at him, he did not seem like a ruler of the people, and approaching him, I still did not see anything that inspires awe."
> (*Mencius* 1A6)

The *Mencius* also seems to think a prince should *sound* like a prince:

> 何其聲之似我君也此無他居相似也
> How is it that his voice is so like that of our prince? This has no other cause than the similarity of their respective positions.[23]
> (*Mencius* 7A36)

In praising the most expressive part of the body, the *Mencius* notes that the pupil is bright or dull in accordance with the alignment of the heartmind in the center.[24] As noted in Chapter 2, the passage is typical of the *Mencius's* frequent pairings of speech and visual manifestation as parallel expressions of their origin.[25] The *Mencius* 3A2, which describes the ordinary custom regarding people in mourning, also pays specific attention to their visual manner and their sound.[26] When the *Mencius* explains the process of understanding, there is a movement, beginning in the heartmind, that extends to both visual expression and sound.[27] In order to dissemble, the body has to struggle. The *Mencius* quotes Confucius's followers as saying,

> 曾子曰脅肩諂笑病于夏畦
> 子路曰未同而言觀其色赧赧然
> Zengzi said, "Shrugging the shoulders and laughing flatteringly is more strenuous than summer fieldwork." Zi Lu said, "When people speak without being in agreement, if you observe their complexions, they are full of blushes." *(Mencius* 3B7)

Thus, it is possible to work against the connection between the heartmind and the periphery of the body, but the *Mencius* expects that some aspect of the person will reveal this struggle.[28] In sum, the *Mencius* seems generally confident that, in terms of a person's heartmind and other features, the "braches" will reflect the "roots." Even in attempts at duplicity, it expects that some features will divulge it.

This confidence in the connection between the heartmind and aural and visual expression results in a difference between the *Mencius's* criteria for reliability and that of the *Xunzi*. Insofar as it pairs vision and sound, the *Mencius* resembles other philosophical texts in the period. However, the *Mencius* actually insists in some places that the two need not correspond. These passages are puzzling, both because the text seems to contradict them elsewhere, and because they are at odds with the "common sense" of the period. However, in light of that common sense position, we can see the uniqueness of the *Mencius* in its peculiar confidence in the heartmind's relation to the periphery of the person. The *Mencius* understands the aural/visual parallels to be rooted in the heartmind, hence it expects them to manifest the heartmind in a reliable manner.

Comparison of the *Laozi* and the *Zhuangzi*

The *Laozi* and the *Zhuangzi* seem to recognize and deliberately critique parts of the shared understanding of the senses in other Warring States philosophical texts. Most obviously, the *Laozi* acknowledges the view that the senses desire excessively, but it challenges common sense in the way that it opts to thwart this tendency. For its part, the *Zhuangzi* clearly recognizes the significance of the eye and ear in producing reliable knowledge, and describes a method of undermining it. Thus, in different ways, both texts reject the standard approach to the senses. This section will focus on an aspect of their respective positions that illuminates the difference between the two texts. That is, both the *Laozi* and the *Zhuangzi* present methods of escaping life's confines and achieving a kind of boundless inexhaustibility. The difference in their methods is manifest in their respective proposals for subverting the ordinary use of the senses. I will argue that in the *Laozi* this is achieved by prohibiting sensory excess, in order to boundlessly expand satisfaction in moderation. In the *Zhuangzi*, on the other hand, this is achieved without recourse to prohibitions, by opening up the senses and clearing them out.

The Laozi

The *Laozi*'s comments on the senses emerge in the context of a critique of desire and a program to escape its exhausting effects.

The *Laozi* seems to view the senses as dangerous because of their tendency to stimulate desire. The *Laozi* implies that the senses' "correlates" present a health hazard—that is, according to the *Laozi*, the sense functions are destroyed by their respective correlates:

> 五色使人目盲
> 馳騁田臘使人心發狂
> 難得之貨使人之行仿
> 五味使人之口爽
> 五音使人之耳聾
> 是以聖人之治也為腹而不為目
> 故去彼而取此
>
> The five colors cause people's eyes to go blind. Riding and hunting cause people's heartminds to go crazy. Goods that are hard to obtain cause people's actions to be obstructed; the five colors cause people's mouths to miss the mark. The five tones cause people's ears to go deaf. Therefore, the sage's government is for the stomach, and not the eye. Thus, he rejects that and takes this.
> (*Laozi* 12)

It is not immediately clear what threat is contained in things like the five colors and tones, or what it means to be "for the stomach, and not the eye." However, the reference to "goods that are hard to obtain" may be a clue. The passage compares the richness of colors, sounds, and tastes with the richness of rare objects and riding and condemns it all. Thus, we may infer that the *Laozi* considers colors, sounds, and tastes to be somehow like rare objects, and rare objects to be somehow like riding and hunting. What all of these items seem to have in common for the *Laozi* may be illuminated by its other comment about riding. In Chapter 46, the *Laozi* connects using racing horses to till the land with knowing how to restrict desire:[29]

> 天下有道卻走馬以糞
> 天下無道戎馬生於郊
> 罪莫大於可欲
> 禍莫大於不知足
> When the world has the way, the racing horses are withdrawn for dung.
> When the world lacks the way, war horses are bred on the borders.
> No crime is greater than being desirable.
> No misfortune is greater than being insatiable.[30]
> (*Laozi* 46)

Hence, riding and hunting stimulate desire, which the *Laozi* condemns along with richness of the senses' desires. This is confirmed by the *Laozi*'s other references to the stomach, wherein the sage empties the heartminds of the people and fills their bellies.

> 是以聖人之治也
> 虛其心實其腹
> 弱其志強其骨
> Therefore, in the government of the sage:
> He empties their heartminds, and fills their bellies,
> Weakens their ambition, and strengthens their bones.
> (*Laozi* 3)

Assuming some consistency between these chapters, the point of being "for the stomach and not the eyes" seems to be that the *Laozi* favors minimizing desires and avoiding stimulating attractions.[31] Along with emptying the heartmind and filling the belly, *Laozi* 3 recommends weakening ambition, while strengthening bones. With a full stomach and strong bones, but little ambition or desire, one is in a position to be hearty, healthy, and content.[32] In other words, pacified senses are not threatening—the senses are only dangerous insofar as they stimulate desires.

Indeed, it is generally apparent that the *Laozi* views desire itself as dangerous. Although there are instances in the *Laozi* of unproblematic desire, in the cases where the *Laozi* explicitly comments on desire, it speaks against it.[33] The *Laozi* associates desire with crime:

> 罪莫大於可欲
> Of crimes—none is greater than being desirable.
> (*Laozi* 46)

According to the *Laozi*, the sage "causes the people to be without knowledge and without desires" (使民無知無欲也, *Laozi* 3). If, however, desires still arise, the sage subdues them:

> 而欲作吾將鎮之
> If desires are created,
> I would subdue them.
> (*Laozi* 37, *Wang Bi* edition)

In some cases, the *Laozi* says that one should merely not desire to the extent of fullness:

> 葆此道者不欲盈
> One who nurtures this way does not desire fullness.
> (*Laozi* 15)

On the same lines, the *Laozi* recommends curtailing desire and reducing self-interest:

> 少私寡欲
> Reduce self-interest and make few your desires.
> (*Laozi* 19, *Wang Bi* edition)

However, in other cases, the *Laozi* advocates being constantly without desire (恆 無 欲 *Laozi* 1 and 34) and desiring not to desire:

> 是以聖人欲不欲
> 而不貴難得之貨
> Therefore, the sage desires not to desire and does not value things that are hard to obtain.[34]
> (*Laozi* 64)

Because the latter prohibition (eliminating all desires) inevitably runs into paradox, we may consider it hyperbolic and follow the former interpretation (viewing the *Laozi* as endorsing minimizing desires). That is, because it is impossible to eliminate *all* desire, we may take the text as simply encouraging the reduction of desire.

But why does the *Laozi* view desire as dangerous? The *Laozi* is clearly not opposed to all forms of physical satisfaction, because it "fills people's bellies" and is "for the stomach." Moreover, it speaks with praise for people who relish simple foods and find beauty in plain clothing (*Laozi* 80, discussed below). If desire's fault is not its physicality, then some other explanation must be sought.

On the basis of what it says about the senses, it seems that the *Laozi* considers desire to be dangerous because of the way it leads to extremes. This is apparent from the *Laozi*'s indictment of extreme forms of sensing—for example, the *Laozi*'s criticism of hearing points to its excess and the exhaustion that results from it:

> 多聞數窮
> 不若守於中
> Much hearing: frequent exhaustion. It is not as good as preserving within.[35]
> (*Laozi* 5)

The *Laozi*'s *dao* itself seems to be restricted in terms of taste, sight, hearing, and "completion." The notion that each of the senses desires to know the fullest of its correlates (as described in Chapter 2) helps explain the *Laozi*'s position here:

> 故道之出言也曰淡呵
> 其無味也
> 視之不足見也
> 聽之不足聞也
> 用之不可既也
> Therefore, of the way's emitting speech, we say:
> Bland! its lack of flavor![36]
> When you look at it, there is not enough to see;
> When you listen to it, there is not enough to hear;
> When you use it, it's not possible to finish.
> (*Laozi* 35)

In other words, its way is deliberately bland, barely visible, and barely heard.

For other evidence of such muted sensory stimuli, we might consider the *Laozi*'s comments about "great images" and "great tones." The *Laozi* refers to these in the context of describing "great squares" and "great vessels," claiming that a great square has no corners, and a great vessel is unfinished:

> 大方無禺大器免成
> 大音希聲天象無刑
> 道褒無名
> 夫唯道善始且善成
> A great square has no corners;
> A great vessel avoids completion;
> A great tone barely sounds;
> A great image lacks form.
> The way is great without a name.
> Only the way is good at beginning and good at completion.
> (*Laozi* 41)

Each of these things is a standard—square, vessel, sound, shape, and way.[37] But each standard lacks something. The example of the vessel not being finished precludes the possibility that the *Laozi* is saying these standards lack their defining characteristics. Moreover, the *Laozi* does not seem to be describing standards that exist in some ideal realm (as it might be if the lines read something like, "There is a great square and it has no corners"). Instead, it seems to be objecting to a certain kind of standard and promoting another kind. The point appears to be that the *Laozi* recommends a standard of incompletion (the vessel example) or a standard that is reversed in some way (the sound example). Although the standard is thus muted in some fashion, according to the last line, this muting is, in fact, the very way to be good at *both* ends of an action—beginning and completion.[38] Thus, the *Laozi*'s depiction of sensory moderation has bearing on its rejection of desire. The senses stimulate desire, and desire leads to excess; therefore, the *Laozi*'s sensory model is moderate or stunted.

The *Laozi*'s frequent prohibition of excess confirms this notion that desire should be avoided as a result of its tendency toward excess. The rejection of excess is a common theme in the text. For example, the sage "dismisses the extreme, the grand, and the excessive" (去甚去大去諸, *Laozi* 29). The *Laozi* says the sage should limit rather than fill, and stop rather than create extremes (sharpen):

> 持而盈不如其已
> 揣而梲之不可長保
> To uphold and fill it,
> Is not so good as ending it.
> If you pound it into a point,
> It won't be preservable for long.
> (*Laozi* 9, *Wang Bi* edition)

Thus, the reason desire is problematic is that it is interminable and leads to exhaustion.

In reaction to the threat of exhaustion presented by excess of sensory desires, the *Laozi* recommends something like a sensory program of non-action. The *Laozi* critiques visual forms of excess, when the sage warns,

> 光而不眺
> Be bright but do not dazzle.
> (*Laozi* 58)

In the context of *dao*, the *Laozi* talks about looking without seeing, listening without hearing, and so on.[39] In the most explicit example, the *Laozi* recommends that the sage "taste without tasting," along with the more familiar *wei wuwei* (act without acting, do without doing, or be for without being for):

> 為無為事無事味無未
> Act without acting;
> Serve without serving;
> Taste without tasting.
> (*Laozi* 63)

Each of these cases involves a two-part action, only one part of which is acted out, the other remaining withheld.[40] The *Laozi*'s metaphor of blocking holes seems to be a variation on this theme of half-performed sensory actions. Although it never explicitly connects the holes to the senses, the association seems justified.[41] In the first case, after mentioning blocking holes, the *Laozi* makes one of its seemingly paradoxical statements of reversal about the senses:

> 塞其兑閉其門 終身不動
> 開其兑濟其事 終身不救
> 見小日明守柔日強

Block up the holes; close the doors;
And till the end of your life you won't work.
Open the holes; meddle in affairs;
And till the end of your life you won't be saved.
Seeing little is called "clarity."
Preserving weakness is called "strength."
(*Laozi* 52, *Wang Bi* edition)

In the second case, prior to mentioning blocking doors, the *Laozi* criticizes speaking (which involves opening the mouth). Moreover, immediately after that, it recommends modulating light and blunting (tactile?) edges:

知者不言言者不知
塞其兑閉其門
挫其鋭解其分
和其光同其塵
One who knows doesn't speak; one who speaks doesn't know.
Block one's holes, close one's doors,
File down one's sharp points, untie one's tangles.
Harmonize one's light, and grind one's dust.
(*Laozi* 56, *Wang Bi* edition)

A similar passage that advises against using doors and windows also advises against seeing:

不出戶知天下
不闚牖見天道
其出彌遠其知彌少
是以聖人
不行而知不見而名不為而成
Don't leave the door, [and yet] know the world;
Don't peer out the window, [and yet] see heaven's way.
The farther you go, the less you know.

Therefore, the sage knows without acting [lit. walking],
Names without seeing,
And completes without doing.[42]
(*Laozi* 47, *Wang Bi* edition)

These hole-blocking metaphors imply that closing off, or at least partially limiting, the senses is the proper way of action. Like the "non-acted" sensory acts described above, these allusions to the senses generally suggest a method of avoiding sensory extremes.[43]

With regard to the senses, the practical application of this half-performed method seems to amount to returning to simple, moderate sensory discriminations. For example, Chapter 80 endorses the value of simple tastes, in the context of small, isolated social units. The passage hints that the senses should be subject to reduction and simplicity:

使人復結繩而用之
甘其食美其服安其居樂其俗
鄰國相望雞犬之聲相聞
民至老死不相往來

Cause the people to return to knotting cords and using them, finding sweet their food, finding beautiful their clothes, finding joyful their customs, finding security in their lodgings.
Nearby states look to one another, the sounds of chickens and dogs hear one another, [yet] the people arrive at old age and die without comings and goings among one another.
(*Laozi* 80, *Wang Bi* edition)

When read in this light, the muted and stunted sensory acts in the rest of the text may be seen as attempts to return to the enjoyment of simple sensory pleasure. Tasting "no taste" and exhibiting brightness without being dazzling might be achieved by appreciating simple foods and clothes. Thus, the danger of desires would be conquered by cutting off sensory pleasure before it reaches an extreme.

The sense reactions of infancy seem to be another metaphor for this blunted form of sensory pleasure. The *Laozi*'s vivid description of the newborn babe, in addition to showing that weakness is strength, establishes an analogy between an infant and one who is full of *de* (charisma/virtue) (Chapter 55). Moreover, the *Laozi* specifically describes the sage as "taking nourishment from the mother" (Chapter 20). Hence, the sage resembles an infant feeding at its mother's breast. At the same time, the eyes and ears of the common people also seem infantile in their lack of agency—while the sage takes their heartmind as his own (adopts their concerns?), the common people "make their eyes and ears belong to him" (屬耳目焉), watching and listening to him alone (Chapter 49). Thus, the non-active tasting, hearing, and seeing recommended by the *Laozi* also appear to be like those of an infant. Presumably the infant, like the simple social beings in Chapter 80, finds satisfaction in its very moderate sensory pleasures.

The shared view in the Warring States philosophical texts that sense–desire is excessive situates the *Laozi*'s program within a larger context. The *Laozi* recognizes the standard view that desire tends to be interminable, unless properly checked. The *Laozi*'s solution of rejecting sensory excess and thereby finding inexhaustible resources for satisfaction is typical of its general theme of non-action. Making the most of the prohibition (the no in not-acting), it restricts and returns to isolated primitive groups (at the social level) or to infancy (at the individual level).

The Zhuangzi

Like the *Laozi*, the *Zhuangzi* reacts against the status quo in its treatment of the senses. However, in the *Zhuangzi*, the senses are not blocked or checked in order to escape danger. Instead, the

Zhuangzi contains many cases of "externalizing," which seems to necessitate opening the senses for circulation. This open model of sensing points to a significant difference between the two texts. In the *Laozi*, the motivation for restricting the senses is grounded in an attempt to avoid desire, because desire leads to excess and exhaustion. The *Laozi* seeks a kind of boundlessness within the context of prohibiting excess of sensory desires—for example, a limitless appreciation of flavor gained by keeping to simple flavors. By contrast, the *Zhuangzi* focuses less on the topic of desire. The *Zhuangzi* also seems less troubled by excess. In the *Zhuangzi*, the senses are open, like hollows and cavities blown about by the wind, and permit access to things like spirits and *qi*. In this way, the senses suggest boundless exposure and boundless freedom. Thus, while the *Laozi* prohibits excess in order to gain boundless freedom from exhaustion, the *Zhuangzi* describes a boundlessness that involves no restrictions. These different subversions of the senses suggest a larger contrast, in which the *Laozi* discovers boundlessness through prohibitions and the *Zhuangzi* discovers it without them.

The *Zhuangzi* associates the senses with spaces that can be open or closed, empty or full. There are a number of ways in which the *Zhuangzi* does this. With the human body as a microcosm of the universe, the *Zhuangzi* calls caves and cavities of the earth nostrils, mouths, ears, and sockets that are piped by the wind:

> 山林之畏佳大木百圍之竅穴
> 似鼻似口似耳似枅
> In the crevices of mountain forests, the hollows from huge trees a hundred spans around are like mouths, like ears, like sockets.
> (*Zhuangzi* 2/5–6)

In addition to labeling these "ten thousand hollows" (萬 竅) of the earth as senses, elsewhere it calls the senses themselves "hollows."

That is, when evaluating the bodily parts, it refers to the senses as "nine hollows" (九竅 2/16). And in the Hun Dun passage, Hun Dun's friends—who want to do him the favor of making him like humans—drill him seven holes that kill him:

> 人皆有七竅以視聽食息此獨無有嘗試鑿之
> 日鑿一竅七日而渾沌死
> Everyone has seven holes in order to look, listen, eat, and breathe. This one alone does not have them. Let us try boring them. Each day they bored one hole and on the seventh day, Hun Dun died.
> (*Zhuangzi* 7/34–35)

Such passages serve to indicate that, for the *Zhuangzi*, the senses are nodal points—holes or openings of the person.

In the *Zhuangzi*, as in the *Laozi*, a number of passages suggest that the sensory openings expose the person to danger. In addition to confirming that the body's senses are holes, the Hun Dun passage cited above also conveys the impression that such holes are dangerous.[44] Moreover, in another passage, the awakened form's openings (*kai* 開) to the world create contacts that "drag" it, and create contention for the heartmind:

> 其寐也魂交
> 其覺也形開
> 與接為搆
> 日以心鬥
> When it is sleeping, the *hun* spirits cross.
> When it wakes, the form opens.
> [Things it] has contact with become pulls [on it].
> Each day we use our heartminds to quarrel.
> (*Zhuangzi* 2/10)

Given that the eyes (and also the ears, in a different way) are closed during sleep, this seems to say that the eyes and ears open when the form awakens and lead the heartmind to quarreling.[45] Thus, opening the senses is a source of trouble.

But in the *Zhuangzi*, this danger posed by the senses being open is framed less in terms of the problem of desire (as in the *Laozi*) than in terms of inappropriate emission or admission. When the *Zhuangzi* discusses holes, there is often a complementary structure wherein something entering (*ru* 入) coincides with something exiting (*chu* 出).[46] For instance, *Zhuangzi* 5/45 (discussed in Chapter 4) says changes of circumstances (like life and death, survival and loss, and so on) should not "enter" the "spiritual residence," while peace and joy should not be lost through openings.[47] On the same lines, in preparation for contact with a dangerous person, one of *Zhuangzi*'s characters suggests rectifying the body, which it depicts as the form approaching without entering, and the heartmind having peace without emitting (*chu* 出) (see *Zhuangzi* 4/56–58, page 105). Thus, the danger of keeping the senses open is that, in accordance with certain things entering, other things like peace and joy might be lost.

In the *Zhuangzi,* the emission of knowledge is a particularly prominent danger posed by opening the senses. The *Zhuangzi* specifically opposes emitting (*chu* 出) knowledge, which it associates with the loss of *de*:

> 且若亦知夫德之所蕩而知之所為出乎哉
> 德蕩乎名知出乎爭
> 名也者相札〔軋〕也
> 知也者爭之器也二者凶器
> 非所以盡行也
>
> Besides, do you after all realize that what dissipates *de* is what activates knowledge to come out? *De* is dissipated over names [fame]. Knowledge is emitted over competition. Names are things that subvert one another. Knowledge is something that is an instrument of struggle.

> The two of them are inauspicious weapons, and not that by which one might perfect one's actions.
> (*Zhuangzi* 4/5–7)

The *Zhuangzi* does not *say* that knowledge is emitted through the use of the eyes and ears, but its injunctions to expel knowledge are often preceded by dismissing the eyes and ears. The *Zhuangzi* rejects the eyes and ears together as a pair four times, and in three of these cases this precedes a rejection of the heartmind or knowledge. The *Zhuangzi* dismisses the eyes and ears of the common people—one of the Mohist criteria for evaluating knowledge (see *Zhuangzi* 6/69–71, page 58). This expelling of the eyes and ears seems to be a precondition for getting rid of knowledge and uniting with a greater current (see *Zhuangzi* 6/92–93, page 58). Along the same lines, the *Zhuangzi* also describes certain sages as dismissing the individual's eyes and ears, and unknowing the starting point for measuring (see *Zhuangzi* 6/69–71 in Chapter 2). Thus, if getting rid of knowledge requires expelling the eyes and ears, it is likely that, ordinarily, the emission of knowledge involves using the eyes and ears. In other words, the *Zhuangzi* seems to be referring to the "tallying knowledge" of the ears and eyes. Hence, a significant cause for concern in opening the senses would be that, as this passage says, *de* is dissipated by the emission of knowledge and, as it implies, the emission of this knowledge takes place through the eyes and ears.

Nevertheless, in spite of these potentially dangerous emissions, the *Zhuangzi* does not propose blocking the sensory holes. Instead of closing the holes, the *Zhuangzi* emphasizes something called "externalizing" (*wai* 外), which seems to require keeping them open.[48] Whereas the *Zhuangzi* criticizes emitting knowledge through the eyes and ears, it speaks positively of externalizing knowledge. As mentioned above, in the *Zhuangzi*, there are many complementary structures involving entering and exiting. In this case, the process of externalizing knowledge seems to be counterpoint to following the inwardly circulating movements of the eyes and ears (see *Zhuangzi* 4/32–33, page 59). To permit the arrival of the ghostly and spiritual (as well as the departure of knowledge), it seems that these inward channels must be open for circulation.[49] In fact, far from closing off communication at the borders of the ears and eyes, the *Zhuangzi* recommends externalizing the bones and body—which amounts to externalizing the eyes and ears themselves.[50] It is not clear what externalizing bones and body actually entails, but it seems to promise liberation beyond all boundaries: Confucius explains that a group of men who externalize their own bones and body (外其形骸) manage to roam outside all direction (*fang* 方), whereas he merely roams inside direction.[51] By "following the channels inward" and "externalizing," the *Zhuangzi*'s characters both roam freely and facilitate communication with the spirits.

The notion that the senses must be left open for the spiritual elements is confirmed by the *Zhuangzi*'s opposition to externalizing the *shen*. This is the one type of externalizing that the *Zhuangzi* explicitly condemns. The *Zhuangzi* criticizes Hui Shi in this way:

> 今子外乎子之神勞乎子之精
> Now you keep on externalizing your *shen* [spirits] and overworking your *jing* [seminal power].
> (*Zhuangzi* 5/59)

Presumably the *shen* comes in through circulating in the senses.[52] In fact, it is not clear whether spiritual things originally belong inside or outside, which is all the more reason to keep open the sensory connections between inside and outside. In any case, as *Zhuangzi* 4/43 indicates, following the currents of the eyes and ears and externalizing knowledge seems to be the way to allow the *shen* to arrive.

The importance of the spiritual aspects for sensing is evident in the only two detailed accounts of sense discrimination in the *Zhuangzi*. One concerns seeing and the other hearing. Both passages mention stopping the ordinary use of the senses.[53] At the point where the ordinary use of the ear and eye stops, the sense is overtaken by what seem to be more tenuous agents. Thus, in place of the eyes, seeing is performed by the *shen*.[54] As Cook Ding describes himself,

> 始臣之解牛之時所見無非牛也
> 三年之後未嘗見全牛也
> 方今之時臣以神遇而不以目視
> 官知止而神欲行依乎天理批大卻
> 導大窾因其固然
> When I first began carving oxen, what I saw was nothing but oxen. After three years, I never saw a complete oxen. Now these days, I use my *shen* to meet [things] and do not look with my eyes. The senses know to stop, and the *shen* desires to go. I follow heaven's pattern, cleave along the main seams, am guided by the main hollows, and rely on what is assuredly so.
> (*Zhuangzi* 3/5–7)

Although perhaps not quite as spiritual as the *shen*, hearing is also overtaken by something equally tenuous—the *qi*. In the "fasting of the heartmind" passage, Confucius instructs Yan Hui not to listen with the ear, but with the *qi*, because it is empty and "awaits." The passage is confusing (the instructions are rather vague, and Confucius simultaneously seems to advocate and oppose listening with the heartmind), but whatever "fasting" might really amount to, the *Zhuangzi* emphasizes the *emptiness* of the *qi*:

> 若一志無聽之以耳而聽之以心
> 無聽之以心而聽之以氣
> 聽止於耳心止於符
> 氣也虛而待物者也
> 唯道集虛虛者心齋也

> Unify your intention. Don't listen with your ears, but listen with your heartmind. Don't listen with your heartmind, but listen with your *qi*. Listening stops at the ear, the heartmind stops at tallying. As for *qi*, it is empty and awaits things. Only the way accumulates emptiness. The emptiness is the heartmind's fasting.
> (*Zhuangzi* 4/26–28)

Unlike the emptying of the heartmind in *Laozi* 3—which coincides with filling the stomach—the tenuousness in these passages is not counterbalanced by filling something else. The *Zhuangzi* has no interest in keeping the common people well fed or in tasting "no-taste" in the sense of relishing simple foods. (The food eaten by the "genuine people" in the *Zhuangzi* is simply not sweet at all—其食不甘, *Zhuangzi* 6/6.)[55] Thus, instead of blocking the senses in order to appreciate their simple pleasures, the *Zhuangzi* seems to be airing them out.

Indeed, whereas the *Laozi* presents the infant and the isolated community as models for proper use of the senses, the *Zhuangzi*'s models seem to be people breathing with their feet and walking on air.[56] Perhaps not arbitrarily, the *Zhuangzi* chooses the loss of a foot as its example of a kind of difference sensed by ordinary use of eyes and ears:

> 自其異者視之肝膽楚越也
> 自其同者視之萬物皆一也
> 夫若然者且不知耳目之所宜
> 而遊心乎德之和物視其所一
> 而不見其所喪視喪其足猶遺土也
>
> Looked at from the viewpoint of their differences, from liver to gall is as far as from Chu to Yue. Looked at from the viewpoint of their sameness, the myriad things are all one. Such people do not even know what is appropriate to the ears and eyes, and they roam their heartminds in the

> peace of *de*. With things, they look at that which makes them one and do not see that which makes their losses. They look at losing their feet like leaving behind the ground.
> (*Zhuangzi* 5/7–8)

As if proving that they do not know what is appropriate to the ears and eyes, the passage notes that these characters look at oneness. Thus, the passage suggests that what *is* appropriate to the ears and eyes is looking at losses, rather than oneness. The example of the loss (*sang* 喪) of a foot—representing the not-oneness sensed by the ears and eyes—may help clarify the use of the senses in the *Zhuangzi*. "Walking" (in the sense of "walk the talk") is the basic metaphor for fulfilling speech and making it accountable.[57] That is, the "appropriate hearing and seeing" depends in part upon being able to see someone walking. In this passage, the walking is lost because the foot is lost. This is a curious pun, because the character for feet (*zu* 足) can also be used to mean the opposite of loss—"enough" or "sufficient." Thus, perhaps this lost foot represents the senses' unfulfillable desire to know satisfaction, as well as knowing what is appropriate to tallying the ears and eyes.

The metaphorical weight of the lost foot is enhanced by the peculiar number of foot references in the *Zhuangzi*. (In Chapter 5, there are three different footless characters, and Confucius compares a dead pig to a footless person. In Chapter 4, a madman is anxious about having his feet wounded.) On the face of it, lost feet refer to crimes that are punished by amputation. However, there were *other* body parts that could be amputated. Furthermore, the *Zhuangzi* also mentions feet even when they are not lost—the old men of old breathe through their heels (in contrast to the common people who talk with their throats), and Huzi's impulses come up from his heels. With all these feet replaced by air, none of these characters are walking on the ground.

Not uncharacteristically, the *Zhuangzi* reverses the value of this "loss" of accountability/enough. This loss—like having the feet filled with breath—is conducive to roaming the mists, seated galloping, and that general sort of thing:

> 絕跡易無行地難....
> 吉祥止止夫且不止是之謂坐馳
> To stop leaving footprints is easy, not walking on the ground is hard....The blessed, the auspicious, stops the stopping. And moreover not stopping—this I call "seated galloping."
> (*Zhuangzi* 4/30–32)

Thus, with this loss, the *Zhuangzi*'s characters are free to talk and walk boundlessly.[58] The *Zhuangzi* replaces the ears' and eyes' "appropriate" measurements of loss with heavenly measurements that balance out differences (thereby producing a kind of oneness like that which corresponds to not knowing what is appropriate to the ears and eyes in *Zhuangzi* 5/7). Defying boundaries in this way, they proceed to "walk in two directions":

> 是以聖人和之以是非而休乎天鈞
> 是之謂兩行
> This is why the sage smoothes things out with "That's it, that's not," and rests on heaven's potter's wheel. This is called "walking in two directions."
> (*Zhuangzi* 2/39–40)

That is, by giving up ordinary hearing and seeing (or "losing the foot"), they acquire footless walking, which is some kind of "unknowing knowing":

> 絕跡易無行地難....聞以有知知者矣
> 未聞以無知知者也

> To stop leaving footprints is easy, not walking on the earth is hard.... You've heard of the knowing that uses knowing. You have not yet heard of the knowing that uses not-knowing.
> (*Zhuangzi* 4/30–32)

This suggests that just as walking with lost feet is unknowing, so too having feet (or having enough) is knowing, in the sense of using the ears and eyes to discriminate differences. By giving up the ears, eyes, and feet/sufficiency, the characters no longer walk on earth and are free to roam on air.

For the *Zhuangzi*, the senses are holes that pose dangers. In particular, the eyes and ears pose the danger of emitting knowledge. The *Zhuangzi* rejects knowledge, yet it does not advise closing off the senses, as the *Laozi* does. The *Zhuangzi* seems to favor keeping the senses open and using the *shen* and *qi* to sense, while unknowing the differences discriminated by the ears and eyes. In a way, the *Zhuangzi* seems to make the ears and eyes more like the nose—empty holes where breath comes in and out. In so doing, it allows both speech and action to extend into the infinite and roam in the boundless.

Conclusions

The contrast between the *Xunzi*'s emphasis on outcomes and the *Mencius*'s emphasis on origins has a particular explanation in reference to sense discrimination. Both texts observe the reliability of correspondence between hearing and vision, but the texts justify that reliability in different ways. True to its concern with outcomes, the *Xunzi* explains aural/visual reliability as the consequence of matching aural and visual responses. By contrast, in keeping with its emphasis on correct origins, the *Mencius* explains aural/visual reliability as the result of shared derivation. In other words, this feature of sense discrimination is treated differently in ways consistent with the differences between these two texts.

The differences between the *Laozi* and the *Zhuangzi* are often obscured by viewing them both as Daoists. This analysis of their treatment of sense discrimination highlights certain contrasts between them. The *Laozi* and the *Zhuangzi* both suggest methods of subverting the ordinary use of the senses, but they do so in different ways. The *Laozi* focuses on desires and recommends prohibiting extremes by closing off the senses. The result is a kind of boundless sensory appreciation of simplicity. For its part, the *Zhuangzi* seems to recommend dismissing the senses' knowledge, as well as opening the senses to all kinds of potential communications. Here too the result is a kind of boundlessness—in this case one that is not connected with simplicity, but with exceeding measurements.

The fact that these different texts take different positions regarding sense discrimination—positions that nevertheless seem to reflect some common underlying assumptions—may confirm the value of this study. That is, one virtue of this analysis may lie in its capacity to shed light on a common view of sense discrimination without presuming that all of the texts agree about all aspects of the subject.

The implications of this study could go beyond what has been described here. The importance of aural and visual pairings may shed light on other frequent pairings in Warring States texts. For instance, aural and visual pairing may also map onto *yue* 樂 (music) and *li* 禮 (ritual *movements*?). Moreover, the aural/visual pairings may even extend beyond these texts and this period. They certainly seem to apply to the pairing of *ming* 名 (title) and *xing* 形 (performance) in the *Han Feizi*. If indeed it is correct to hypothesize that *shi* 實 is a visual pair for *ming* 名 in these texts, in the future, scholars may find it worth investigating how and when Chinese ontology altered, such that *shi* comes to be used to mean something more like "substance" and "reality."

Notes

Introduction

1. The term "sense discrimination" (as opposed to "sense perception" or "sensation") is chosen for its relative lack of specific philosophical connotations (see Chapter 1). By "sense," I mean things like hearing and seeing, and other specialized forms of interaction between the inside and outside of a human being (not necessarily on the surface of the body). By "discrimination," I mean the general operations characteristic of each of the senses.

2. By "heartmind" I mean the character *xin* 心, the translation of which is discussed below.

3. The term "early China" often includes the Qin dynasty (221 B.C.E.–206 B.C.E.) and the Han dynasty (206 B.C.E.–220 C.E.); however, this study does not extend beyond the Warring States.

4. By the "history of western metaphysics," I mean to refer to the dominant tradition of metaphysics, as it grew from Greek, Jewish, and Christian thought and developed in Western Europe. The phrasing is not meant to imply that the tradition does not include heterogeneous elements that challenge the dominant mode.

5. These were not schools in the sense of institutions. Nathan Sivin argues convincingly against such a notion of an "academy" in early China. Nathan Sivin, "The Myth of the Naturalists," in *Medicine, Philosophy, and Religion in Ancient China* (Brookfield, Vt.: Variorum, 1995), 19–28.

6. As far as can be ascertained, organizing texts into schools began only with a bibliographer in the second century B.C.E. A. C. Graham describes this development as it appears in the work of Sima Tan (d. 110 B.C.E.) and a late chapter of the *Zhuangzi*. A. C. Graham, *Disputers of the Tao: Philosophical Argumentation in Ancient China* (LaSalle, Ill.: Open Court, 1989), 376.

7. A great many archaeological discoveries, occurring over the course of this century, have radically changed traditional understandings of early Chinese history. The trend to interpret classical Chinese philosophical texts as layered accretions or accumulations is just one aspect of the new historiography developing in sinology. See, for example, the work of Bruce and Taeko Brooks. Bruce Brooks and Taeko Brooks, *The Original Analects: Sayings of Confucius and His Successors* (New York: Columbia University Press, 1998).

8. We cannot expect the texts to exhibit the degree of internal coherence and consistency that single authorship is often thought to guarantee. Recognition of multiple authorship may even be a boon, because it liberates interpretation from any attempt to reconstruct the fixed ideas present in the author's mind at the one moment of writing's conception. Instead, we can attempt to reconstruct how the language in these texts functioned in the general historical period.

9. I take the first half of this characterization of "philosophy" from Joel Kupperman's argument for including thinkers like Confucius as philosophers. Joel Kupperman, *Learning from Asian Philosophy* (Oxford: Oxford University Press, 1999), 13. The reference to ethical and political reform I derive from Nathan Sivin's argument that rejects the idea that Chinese thinkers should be evaluated in terms of a modern definition of philosophy. Sivin, *Medicine, Philosophy, and Religion in Ancient China,* 13.

(The *Zhuangzi* counts in this sense, because, although it parodies the desire for ethical and political reform, it does engage the question.) By calling these texts philosophical, I do not mean to imply that they are not religious. Neither category applies very well to early Chinese thought, which is one of the limitations of these categories.

10. Actually, I accept Donald Davidson's principle that cross-cultural understanding cannot avoid presuming that *most* beliefs of the other language/culture are similar to our own. This still leaves plenty of room for difference and error within the kinds of theories we generate. Donald Davidson, *Inquiries into Truth and Interpretation* (Oxford: Clarendon Press, 1984).

11. "Comparison requires the postulation of difference as the grounds of its being interesting (rather than tautological), and a methodological manipulation of difference, a playing across the 'gap' in the service of some useful end." Jonathan Z. Smith, *Imagining Religion: From Babylon to Jonestown* (Chicago: University of Chicago Press, 1982), 35.

12. Ben-Ami Scharfstein, "The Contextual Fallacy," in *Interpreting across Boundaries: New Essays in Comparative Philosophy*, ed. Gerald James Larson and Eliot Deutsch (Princeton: Princeton University Press, 1988), 86.

13. The former was proposed by Xenophanes (c. 343–355 B.C.E.), and the latter by Empedocles (c. 440 B.C.E.).

14. Dallas Willard summarizes this in "Predication as Originary Violence," in Dallas Willard, *Working through Derrida*, ed. Gary B. Madison (Evanston, Ill.: Northwestern University Press, 1993), 120–136.

15. Jacques Derrida, *Writing and Difference* (Chicago: University of Chicago Press, 1978), 279.

16. In speaking of early Chinese 'metaphysics,' I do not mean to imply that the period is characterized by a study of categories of reality or being (like attributes, properties, mind, and possible worlds) or issues of truth (as opposed to justification and warrant). I mean the term in the broad sense that includes cosmology and cosmogony, as well as ontology.

17. Bertrand Russell, *The History of Western Philosophy* (New York: Simon and Schuster, 1945), 45.

18. Continual change should not be taken to mean that everything is always changing in every possible respect, but simply that no thing remains eternally unchanged.

19. This is not to deny the organismic qualities of Greek philosophy. Certainly there are organismic aspects to the cosmologies of Plato and Aristotle (as Donald Munro notes), but in seeking permanent foundational substances, their cosmologies are not organismic. Donald Munro, ed., *Individualism and Holism: Studies in Confucian and Taoist Values* (Ann Arbor, Mich.: The University of Michigan Center for Chinese Studies, 1985), 263.

20. Munro, *Individualism and Holism: Studies in Confucian and Taoist Values*, 263.

21. Frederick Mote, *Intellectual Foundations of China* (New York: Alfred A. Knopf, 1971).

22. Tu Wei-ming, in "The Continuity of Being," in *Confucianism and Ecology: The Interrelation of Heaven, Earth, and Humans*, ed. Mary Evelyn Tucker and John Berthrong

(Cambridge, Mass: Harvard University Center for the Study of World Religions, 1998).

23. Chang describes early Chinese civilization as one of continuity between a number of things, including nature and culture. Kwang-chih Chang, "Ancient China and its Anthropological Significance," in *Archeological Thought in America*, ed. C. C. Lamberg-Karlovsky (Cambridge: Cambridge University Press, 1989), 165. The implications of this are highly controversial for interpretations of Warring States thought. Most understandings of the *Xunzi* (particularly with regard to what is taken to be its views on "human nature" versus ritual) rely heavily on a nature/culture opposition. The work of Edward Machle is a notable exception. According to Machle's reading of the *Xunzi*, culture is not "unnatural"—it is the growth that perfects what we are born with (nature?), which is incapable of ordering itself. Machle seems to think positions of the *Zhuangzi* and the *Laozi* come closer to a nature/culture (*physis/techne*) divide, but his description of that divide sounds more like elite culture versus simple culture. Edward J. Machle, *Nature and Heaven in the Xunzi*, Series in Chinese Philosophy and Culture (Albany: State University of New York Press, 1993), 15.

24. Donald Harper, "Warring States Philosophy and Occult Thought," in *The Cambridge History of Ancient China: From the Origins of Civilization to 221 B.C.*, ed. Michael Loewe and Edward L. Shaughnessy (Cambridge: Cambridge University Press, 1999), 831–832.

25. In the fourth and third centuries B.C.E.., the *Yi* was not yet interpreted in terms of broken and unbroken lines, which more clearly signify the polar relations epitomized by *yin/yang*.

26. Keightley argues that this, in addition to the absence of any great early Chinese mythic confrontation with death (along the lines of characters like Gilgamesh or Achilles), suggests that death was not viewed as a tremendous rupture in the early Chinese world. David N. Keightley, "Early Civilization in China," in *Heritage of China*, ed. Paul S. Ropp (Berkeley: University of California Press, 1990), 34.

27. Thus, Edward Shaughnessy writes, "by emphasizing different aspects of the images, the *Zhou Yi* shows that they...were subject to constant change." Edward L. Shaughnessy, "Western Zhou History," in *The Cambridge History of Ancient China: From the Origins of Civilization to 221 B.C.*, 341.

28. According to the *LiJi* 47/14, the ghost souls remain underground, while the spirit souls ascend.

29. Keightley, *Heritage of China*, 19.

30. Keightley, *Heritage of China*, 28.

31. Donald Harper notes that in the older explanation, which persisted along with the new one, demons and naturalistic pathogens from the outside invaded the body, causing it to malfunction. Donald Harper, "Warring States Philosophy and Occult Thought," in *The Cambridge History of Ancient China: From the Origins of Civilization to 221 B.C.*, 874–883.

32. David Chidester describes a cliché in cultural studies going back to the nineteenth century that says Hebraic culture is fundamentally "auditory," while Greek culture is fundamentally "visual." David Chidester *Word and Light: Seeing, Hearing and Religious Discourse* (Urbana: University of Illinios Press, 1992).

33. See discussion of *Zhuangzi* 7/32 in Chapter 3.

34. I am specifically referring to "speech," rather than "language." I translate the character *yan* 言 as "speech" and *ming* 名 as "names." Early Chinese theories regarding these terms should not be misconstrued as theories about language per se, primarily because language, as a concept, tends to evoke notions of representation and a gap between the real thing designated and the inessential designation. From the perspective of a contemporary "linguistic turn" that critiques these metaphysical notions, the early Chinese theories regarding things like names and speech must be understood as pre-metaphysical. This point is well made by Hans Georg Möller. Moreover, he is certainly right to point out that the linguistic realm in early China is discussed in terms of tensions between a variety of elements, which makes it difficult to isolate from among them something that functions as language. Hans Georg Möller, "The Chinese Theory of Forms and Names (*Xingming Zhi Xue*) and Its Relation to a 'Philosophy of Signs,'" *Journal of Chinese Philosophy* 24: 184–189.

The complex subject of the status of writing in relation to these aural/visual parallels is beyond the scope of this monograph. I hope to address it in future publications.

35. For example, Graham explains *shi* as "solid," "concrete," and "real." Graham, *Disputers of the Tao*, 140.

Chapter One: An Overview of Sense Discrimination

1. The reader should be aware that a significant portion of the evidence for what I take to be the general view of the senses comes from one text—the *Xunzi*—because this is where most of the discussion of the senses occurs. Where the *Xunzi* seems to speak uncontroversially, and where there is no overt or subtle sign of disagreement from other texts, I often take the *Xunzi*'s view to represent the general view.

2. I use the term "senses," rather than "sense organs," because the senses do not always seem to correspond to physical organs, although they are sometimes identified with them.

According to John Hay, "Organs, as discrete physical objects, barely exist in traditional Chinese medical theory....Instead, it identifies functions." Hay describes the early Chinese view of the body parts as orbs and para-orbs that are "enfoldments" of energy. John Hay, "The Body as Microcosmic Source," in *Self as Body in Asian Theory and Practice*, ed. Thomas P. Kasulis (Albany: State University of New York Press, 1993), 187.

3. Actually, there are surprisingly few references to "the five senses" within the texts I am considering. The term occurs twice in the *Xunzi*. (It also occurs twice in the external chapters of the *Zhuangzi*, which are not considered in this study, because traditionally they have been thought to be of a later date.)

4. By the Han Dynasty, this develops into a formalized concept of "five processes" (*wu xing* 五 行), which refer to the phases of the cosmos as a whole. Groups of five are much more significant in the Han, but they are manifest in Warring States texts as well. For instance, see *Laozi* 12, cited in Chapter 3. Graham proposes that groups of five, epitomized by the "five processes," originally related to the four seasons and directions (adding one for the middle); see Graham, *Disputers of the Tao*. Chad Hansen suggests that the five fingers and toes, or the senses themselves, are a more plausible origin (personal communication). It is perhaps useless to speculate which is the most originary form of fives. But the fact that even in early China there are other important systems of 'fives' deserves mention in the context of understanding the five senses.

5. The five colors are green, red, yellow, white, and black. The five flavors are sweet, bitter, salty, sour, and pungent. The five tones, according to Joseph Needham, originally differentiated things like pitch and timbre. Joseph Needham, ed. *Science and Civilization in China* (Cambridge: Cambridge University Press, 1954–), vol. 4, part 1:140–141.

6. In some of the texts, there is an unfortunate dearth of lists of the senses. In fact, no list of four or more senses appears at all in the *Lunyu*, or the so-called inner chapters of the *Zhuangzi*. Arguably, there is one case in the *Laozi* (Chapter 12).

7. As noted earlier, the term *xin* 心 is translated as "heartmind," because cognition and emotion both stem from this function.

Some of these lists of senses include the heartmind as if it were a sensory function. The implications of this are discussed in Chapter 3.

8. It is worth noting that there were not always five senses in Western traditions. Constance Classen argues that five became the proper number after some uncertainty caused by Plato's inclusion of things like hot and cold among the senses, in response to which Aristotle aligned the senses with the five elements. Constance Classen, *Worlds of Sense: Exploring the Senses in History and across Cultures* (London: Routledge, 1993), 2.

9. The *Mozi* says,

手足口鼻耳
從事於義必為聖人
When hands, feet, mouth, nose, and ears are employed for righteousness, then one will surely be a sage.
(*Mozi* 47/20)

10. See *Xunzi* 23/25–26 cited in Chapter 3, along with other examples where the difference goes beyond mere variation in the identity of the fifth sense.

11. *Xunzi* 19/8.

12. *Xunzi* 22/83.

13. *Xunzi* 21/14.

14 "Heaven" is not an ideal translation. The term *tian* 天 refers to heaven, the sky, the ancestors, and/or a personal presence with a will of its own. Insofar as it is differentiated from earth, *tian* is above and sometimes dominant, but it is not transcendent. Moreover, in the *Xunzi*, the term "heaven" often seems to be a synecdoche for "heaven and earth"—the powers of the cosmos, loosely associated with ancestor ghosts and spirits who dwell above and below.

This term "heavenly officers" occurs six times in the *Xunzi*, but not elsewhere in these Warring States philosophical texts. We might take the reference to "heavenly" to mean the "higher" faculties, but the text does not mention that they are higher than anything else. In fact, it describes them as subservient to the heartmind. After introducing things like desires and aversions as "heavenly," *Xunzi* 17/12 introduces the senses as "heavenly officers" and then notes that the heartmind rules over the (other?) senses. Hence, perhaps the *tian* in *tianguan* should be understood as simply meaning "natural."

15. The subject of proper governing is even indirectly evident in the *rejection* of the importance of governing expressed in the *Zhuangzi*.

16. *Xunzi* 22/46 uses another government metaphor for the senses—a puzzling line that praises someone for refraining from "governing" (*zhi* 治) the eyes and ears of the onlookers. It is possible that the character is the result of a scribal mistake.

17. See also *Xunzi* 1/47 and 11/79. The clearest cases of this are in the *Xunzi*, but references to the eyes' and ears' excesses (as in *Mozi* 36/18) also seem to place agency in the senses themselves. The same phenomenon occurs with the senses' knowing (see below).

18. *Se* 色 is a term that functions to mean "color," "face," "appearance," and, by extension, "sexual desire."

19. *Mencius* 6A7; *Mozi* 32/2–3. Comparable comments appear in the *Lunyu* and the *Zhuangzi*. While not mentioning desire per se, Confucius indicts the ubiquity of desire for *se* 色 (see tnote 18), (*Lunyu* 9/18). The *Zhuangzi* 5/57 implies that preferences and aversions constitute the human disposition or condition, although it does not explicitly connect them to the senses.

20. *Xunzi* 23/26; *Mencius* 7B24.

21. The basis of the *Mozi*'s objection is that, when rulers indulge their desires, the people are deprived of fundamental needs:

> 且夫仁者之為天下度也非為其目之所美耳之所樂口之所甘身體之所安以此虧奪民衣食之財仁者弗為也
>
> Moreover, the way that benevolent people treat the world is not for the sake of the beauty of the eyes, the joy/music of the ears, the sweetness of the mouth, or the comfort of the body. By means of these the masses are deprived of

> their materials for clothing and food, thus benevolent people are not motivated by such things.
> (*Mozi* 32/2–3)

22. These two threats posed by sensory desires may also account for the *Mencius*'s warning against the danger of being unfilial through following the desires of the ears and eyes. According to the *Mencius*, the fourth form of unfilial behavior is

> 從耳目之欲以為父母戮
> following the desires of one's ears and eyes, so as to bring one's parents to disgrace.
> (*Mencius* 4B30)

See also *Mozi* 35/38–39 and *Mozi* 37/16–17.

23. This passage (*Zhuangzi* 2/17) does not refer to the senses per se.

24. The wind plays a role in hearing, smelling, and eating (tasting?). It is less clear whether, and to what extent, the wind contributes to other sense functions (like seeing).

25. In the Warring States period, *qi* denotes a very basic component of most things. Eventually, perhaps as early as late Warring States, it is viewed as a component of *all* things. (See the Introduction for discussion of *qi*.)

For its part, *de* seems to function as "charisma," "power," or "virtue," in the sense of what someone (or something—the *Lunyu* 14/33 speaks of a horse's *de*) excels at. By extension, *de* often connotes moral virtue in Warring States texts. However, it is not limited to this usage: *de* can be good or bad, noble or petty. The analysis of *de* here is particularly focused on identifying its more concrete usages, because the topic under consideration is how *de* can be sensed through music.

26. As Shigehisa Kuriyama notes, the Shang divination inscriptions asked questions like, "Will the wind come from the east?" and "Will destructive winds arrive?" Kuriyama also contends that the winds of the four directions were each associated with a divinity. Shigehisa Kuriyama, "The Imagination of Winds," in *Body, Subject, and Power in China*, ed. Angela Zito and Tani Barlow (Chicago: University of Chicago Press, 1994), 33–34.

27. This first line is a visual pun—the desire for the sound of music is so acute that the term for 'music' (*yue* 樂) also functions as the term for 'joy' (*le* 樂).

28. It is surprisingly rare to find mention of the *qi* of specific things. There are only a few references to human and animal *qi* and *qi* of various features of the natural world (see Introduction).

29. The *Zhuangzi* describes the pipes of the earth, saying,

> 夫大塊噫氣其名為風
> The great clump of earth blows out *qi*, whose name is "wind."
> (*Zhuangzi* 2/4)

Kuriyama maintains that *qi* and *feng* are freely substituted for one another in late Warring States texts. Kuriyama, *Body, Subject, and Power in China*, 34.

30. The resonance of sound is not necessarily musical—a similar aural *qi* stimulus, caused by the cry of a dying animal, also stimulates a response in the heartmind:

獸死不擇音氣息茀然於是並生心厲
剋核大至則必有不肖之心應之
When an animal is dying, it does not select its sound: its *qi* and breath are vicious. Thereupon, this causes a mutual birth of fierceness in the heartmind. When subduing and pressuring reaches too far, then you necessarily have the response of a degenerate heartmind.
(*Zhuangzi* 4/50–51)

The sound of an animal seems to be identified with its *qi* and breath. This sound-*qi* also causes the birth of something in the heartmind, which (by analogy in the last line) is its "response."

31. The term *jie* frequently applies to the senses in the *Xunzi*. The *Xunzi* uses the term to explain how sensory desires obstruct thinking:

耳目之欲接則敗其思...
When the desires of the ears and eyes make contact, the thoughts are lost...
(*Xunzi* 21/62)

See also *Xunzi* 17/11 in Chapter 1.

32. Using similar terminology, the *Mencius* describes how sensory contact precludes thinking:

耳目之官不思而蔽於物
物交物則引之而已矣
Thinking is not the office of the eyes and ears, and they are clouded by things. Things interact with things, and pull them astray. That is all.
(*Mencius* 6A15)

Qi is small enough that it may enter the person via the pores in the skin, which are not explicitly included as senses in these texts, except perhaps as "skin lines" (*fuli* 膚理) in *Xunzi* 23/26.

33. The *Zhuangzi* contains one passage that gives some, albeit vague, sense of the relation between *de* and *qi*. A fictitious Confucius tells a fictitious Yan Hui,

> 且德厚信矼未達人氣
> 名聞不爭未達人心
> Furthermore, to be ample in *de* and solid in trustworthiness is not yet to reach someone's *qi*. To be heard in name/reputation as noncompetitive is not yet to reach someone's heartmind.
> (*Zhuangzi* 4/7)

The passage implies that, although possessing these qualifications is not sufficient for achieving such goals, they do contribute to them. Thus, having ample *de* does help bring one close to affecting someone's *qi*. Given that the same can be said of "trustworthiness," it is probably a mistake to infer much more about *de* and its relation to *qi* from this passage.

34. Interestingly, in two instances, water metaphors are employed to portray this accumulation (*Xunzi* 27/84 and *Zhuangzi* 5/ 46).

35. The *Xunzi* describes this process:

> 雨小漢故潛夫盡小者大積微者著
> 德至者色澤洽行盡而聲問遠
> When rain is small, the Han becomes hidden. Something that exhausts the small becomes big; something that

> accumulates the minute becomes manifest. When *de* arrives [reaches completion], the face becomes glossy. When one's actions are exhausted, one is heard from afar. (*Xunzi* 27/83–84)

The *wen* 問 (ask) is regularly emended to be *wen* 聞 (hear).

On the subject of accumulating, perhaps it is significant for the relation of *de* to *qi* that *qi* also fills out the body in *Mencius* 2A2 (氣 體 之 充 也).

36. Stripped of its New Age connotations, "spirit" is an adequate translation for *shen*. *Shen* is often paired with ghost (*gui* 鬼), its earthly counterpart. Although working with material from later periods, in "The Spirits of Chinese Religion," Stephen F. Teiser reconstructs how the term was used. As Teiser explains it, in death, *shen* and *gui* indicate the more or less light, benevolent souls (*hun* 魂) and the denser, malevolent souls (*po* 魄) of dead ancestors. But *shen* has other connotations as well. Teiser breaks the term into three aspects: (1) one's psyche (*hun*), (2) "spirits" in the sense of nontranscendent gods, and (3) something numinous that exceeds categorization. Stephen F. Teiser, "The Spirits of Chinese Religion," in *Religions of China in Practice,* ed. Donald S. Lopez, Jr. (Princeton: University of Princeton Press, 1996), 34–36.

37. I treat *de* and tone as two separate but related things, instead of reading *de* as modifying tone, because of the parallel items in the passage, which are not adjectives modifying nouns.

38. Munro takes a different perspective on the sensory background of *de*, which, he argues, has visual roots in the Western Zhou. Donald Munro, "The Origin of the Concept of *De*," in *The Concept of Man in Early China* (Stanford: Stanford University Press, 1969), 185–197.

39. Of course, some *de* can be harmful instead of beneficial. *Xunzi* 11/77, for example, mentions aberrant and alienating *de*.

40. For some reason, here—as opposed to *Zhuangzi* 2/4—the *Zhuangzi* contrasts wind and *qi*. It notes that riding on wind remains dependent, while riding on *qi* does not.

41. The term *wen* has a dual sense of both hear and smell in later Chinese texts. This is the only instance in these Warring States philosophical texts that hints that *wen* might function as "smell." The rarity may make "hear" a more likely translation.

42. A color patch is one possible example of what counts as sense data, but there is less agreement about the identity of sense data than there is about the definition of the term. D. W. Hamlyn, *Sensation and Perception* (London: Routledge and Kegan Paul, Ltd., 1961), 175.

43. Some forms of representational realism argue that sense data are "given" (immediately known) and independent of the mind's judgment. Wilfred Sellars terms this "the myth of the given" in *Empiricism and the Philosophy of Mind.*

Sellars refutes this view of foundational sensory knowledge by contending that, insofar as someone can claim to have a noninferential, nonverbal belief that s/he is seeing the color red, s/he can only do so in the context of connecting that belief with a network of other understood beliefs. As a result, even if there are noninferential beliefs like the belief that one is seeing red, there is no way for a noninferential belief alone to justify a belief that has conceptual content. Wilfred Sellars, *Empiricism and the Philosophy of Mind* (Cambridge: Harvard University Press, 1997).

44. Sense data are usually thought to provide an immediate foundation of knowledge from which perception derives. However, it is also possible to argue that sensation and perception operate via different functions. Nicholas Humphrey argues for the latter perspective. Nicholas Humphrey, *A History of the Mind* (London: Chatto & Windus, 1992).

45. Ludwig Wittgenstein, *Philosophical Investigations,* 3rd ed., trans. G.E.M. Anscombe (New York: Macmillan, 1958), 193–214.

46. Wittgenstein says, "Is it a question of both seeing and thinking? or an amalgam of the two, as I should like to say?" Wittgenstein, *Philosophical Investigations*, 197.

47. This is not to say that the texts consider the senses invariably reliable. For in that case, the constant tallying of what is heard and seen (described in Chapter 2) would not be necessary. Here I am simply denying that the texts exhibit full-blown sense skepticism (see discussion of *Xunzi* 21/70 below).

48. For instance, when blind people are described as picking out "white" from "black," "white" and "black" do not modify certain things. They *are* the things being picked (see examples in Chapter 4).

In this sense, the language of aspect perception is a little misleading, because one is tempted to think that aspects are aspects *of* some neutral thing. Perhaps it would be clearer to say that colors, shapes, and sounds are "aspect-things."

49. *Xunzi* 2/40 and 4/44–45. I rely on the *Xunzi* here because the other texts do not provide general descriptive terms for how the senses act as a group.

50. For example, in *Xunzi* 21/68–69, the passage does not begin by describing what is "out there." In other words, it does not begin by saying, "There is a tree." Instead, it starts out by saying that *a person sees* a tree.

51. Graham contrasts the realism in these texts to linguistic relativism. In explaining the position in the *Zhuangzi*, Graham writes, "What the thinking...is trying vainly to pin down in words is objectively there...he has to accept it as given." *Disputers of the Dao,* 194.

My argument is different, in that it emphasizes that the senses, as well as names, make discriminations (*bian* 辨). Because the senses also discriminate (and because they tend to do so in terms of desires and aversions), there seems to be an element of human signification in sense discrimination. In that case, names are not uniquely representative of social construction. Thus, names would not be solely at fault for the relativistic effects of social convention. In fact, social convention does not seem to be the cause of relativism. Instead, the instability of perspective (and therefore the instability of standards) seems to be the source of relativistic concerns. Thus, the contrast to realism in these texts is not linguistic relativism, any more than it is idealism or nominalism.

52. Another interpretation would be, "if the five officials record them, but the heartmind does not know them." But that would require supplying new subjects simply because the claim sounds odd as it stands. In fact, in these texts, there are other references to the senses knowing, as well as references to the heartmind speaking (more on the latter in Chapter 3).

53. Some commentators consider this *shuo* 說 to be "explain," a less common use of the character.

54. The *Zhengming* differentiates between two words—*zhi* 知 and *zhi* 智—which Knoblock takes to be a distinction between mere awareness, which is characteristic of all sentient beings, and knowledge, which comes from experience and facts (Knoblock, *Xunzi: A Translation and Study of the Complete Works*, 3:123). Knoblock claims to find support for this distinction in Graham's reading of the Neo-Mohist Canons. But Graham actually discusses the terms differently. He notes a distinction between a *faculty* of knowledge (which he sometimes calls awareness) and its *use*, which, unlike the faculty itself, is capable of error. Thus, unlike Knoblock, Graham is not discussing a distinction between simple, animal awareness and experience-based knowledge.

The distinction in the *Zhengming* passage sounds like a distinction between the means of knowing that are in people and knowledge being united with something:

> 所以知之在人者謂之知
> 知有所合謂之智
> Of the means of knowing, those that are in people [*zai ren zhe*]: we call *zhi* [knowing?].
> Knowledge having its union: we call *zhi* [understanding?].
> (*Xunzi* 22/5)

The section appears to be describing the "assorted names" that can be "applied to people"—*zai ren zhe* 在人者—as opposed to the ten thousand things. The phrase *zai ren zhe* appears repeatedly in the section. It seems to emphasize aspects of things that are located within people. Thus, in the case of knowledge, the first line seems to refer to those means of knowing that are located in people. This would include intelligence among other things and certainly need not be restricted to awareness. I owe this insight to Dan Robins (personal communication).

55. The *Xunzi* uses this unusual term without explanation (see below).

56. Some commentators emend *yi* 疑 to *ni* 擬, but this does not seem to account for the *zhi* 之 following *bifang* 比 方, which I take to be possessive.

57. The agent of this action is unclear, but while it could be any given individual, the larger context is still about how good rulers would rectify names.

58. Later the chapter explains that the rulers affix the names to what they name, suggesting that the affixed names then evolve into habit or custom.

59. Knoblock, *Xunzi* 3:129. Graham initiated the proposal that in some cases *qing* should be understood as "essence" (sometimes in the sense of what a thing must have in order to be called that thing, other times in the sense of "genuine" as opposed to "demeanor"). A. C. Graham, "The Mencian Theory of Human Nature," in *Studies in Chinese Philosophy and Philosophical Literature*, Series in Chinese Philosophy and Culture (Albany: State University of New York Press, 1990), 59–65. "Essence" is not a good translation, however, both because there is little evidence to connect *qing* to a difference between necessary and sufficient conditions for naming things and because it places enormous philosophical weight on *qing* in contexts, such as this one, where the term seems to have no such significance.

The translation of the term *qing* in early China is controversial, because the term is perceived to suggest, on the one hand, objectivity, nature, and reality, and on the other, subjectivity, emotion, and desire. One way to resolve this is to say that some desires derive from reality (as opposed to convention), hence *qingyu* 情 欲 would refer to real desires, as opposed to conventional desires. For example, see Chad Hansen, "*Qing* 情 in Pre-Buddhist Chinese Thought," *Emotions in Asian Thought: A Dialogue in Comparative Philosophy* (Albany: State University of New York Press, 1995), 201. My position is that *qing* is used to connote the feelings and emotions with which we are born, and which comprise the human disposition. They are genuine in the sense of being present (particularly at birth)—and not "awaiting" (*dai* 待) things, as the *Xunzi* frequently says of sensory desires, and *Xunzi* 23/26 specifically says of the *qingxing* (*qing*-nature). Hence, when *qing* is sometimes used to imply genuineness in these texts, this involves a contrast between things that are present and things that are not (or that await development). This can, in some cases, amount to equating human artifice with disingenuousness (as in the case of *qingwei* 情 偽 in *Mozi* 36/2), but it is not *necessarily* a contrast between nature and human convention, because nature also contains things that await (natural) development, as the persistent use of root and sprout metaphors in these texts reminds us.

The association of *qing* with the senses does not render *qing* real or factual, in contrast to convention. Like the *Xunzi,* the *Mozi* also refers to *qing* in the context of the senses. In order to settle doubts, the *Mozi*'s recommends, among other things, consulting the eyes and ears of the common people. The *Mozi* asks,

> 惡乎原之
> 察眾之耳目之請
> How are they to be originated? They are to be checked by the *qing* of the eyes and ears of the multitude.
> (*Mozi* 37/4)

In the *Mozi*, the eyes and ears of the common people are one of three criteria for creating standards for judgments (also including usefulness and the practices of the sage kings). While the *qing* of the eyes and ears plays this important role in the *Mozi*, unlike reality or the facts, *qing* is not indubitable. For example, *Mozi* 31/44 seriously entertains the objection that a gentleman should not deign to follow *qing* from the eyes and ears of commoners. Having acknowledged the role of social rank in deciding a matter, the passage concedes that even the gentleman should follow the eyes and ears of the commoners; however, he should do so only because they concur with what is written about the sage kings. If the critics and the Mohists took the *qing* of the ears and eyes to indicate reality, they would be unlikely to raise this criticism or respond with this concession.

Moreover, the passage says nothing about the *qing* being reliable due to its derivation in the senses, as opposed to human convention. Instead, it implies that the *qing* of the multitude is only as compelling as the multitude, which is not as compelling as the sage kings. The association of *qing* with the senses does not confer on it the persuasiveness of something certain—such as facts or reality. Thus, it seems more likely that the *qing* of the senses are their feelings or dispositions, which are genuine (in the sense that they are immediate and do not await things), but are not as incontrovertible as facts and reality.

For other viewpoints on the translation of *qing*, see Anthony Yu, *Rereading the Stone: Desire and the Making of Fiction in* Dream of the Red Chamber (Princeton: Princeton University Press, 1997), 56–66; and Ong-cho Ng, "Is Emotion (*Qing*) the Source of A Confucian Antimony?", *Journal of Chinese Philosophy* 25: 169–190.

60. For example, Knoblock's translation reads, "Whenever things belong to the same category of being or have the same essential characteristics, the *representation* of them presented by the senses is the same." Knoblock, *Xunzi* 3:129.

61. For a more detailed version of this argument, see my "Mencius's Hermeneutics," *Journal of Chinese Philosophy* 27: 93–100.

62. I take *zi jian* to fit the model in *Xunzi* 21/46–47—"see by themselves." That is, in this circumstance, the dancer's own eyes and ears do not see and hear it, but someone else's might. The point seems to be that the dancer's own eyes and ears are not controlling the order that emerges.

63. *Mencius* 6A15 suggests something like this movement—it compares the senses to things that are tugged (*yin* 引) by other things.

64. Although *Xunzi* 21/70 begins by stating the importance of keeping the heartmind settled, the heartmind is far from the only thing that causes sensory doubts in the passage. As I argue below, an unsettled heartmind is simply one among many unreliable standards, like darkness, distance, and blindness.

65. This could be the number "one" or a single thing.

66. This *hong* is traditionally read as a mistake for a character with a different radical, meaning "uproar." There is a very similar *mo* that means "silence," but it does not have this radical. (This *mo* is commonly translated as "desert.") Watson translates the line as "dull noises will sound like a sharp din" (Watson, *Hsun Tzu*, 134), and Knoblock says "silence seem[s] like a clamor," (Knoblock, *Xunzi*, 3:109). Because both *mo* and *hong* are emended to produce this reading, I do not follow them. Perhaps the point is simply that the words *mo* and *hong* sound different.

67. An earlier line in the passage refers to mistakes in seeing due to darkness, but these particular lines focus on looking and listening.

68. It may be significant that other, less controllable, forms of sense discrimination do not have special terms to indicate the effort of using the sense. That is, there is no effort term in English or Chinese to apply to, say, the attempt to smell or taste. (The relation of feel to touch might count.)

69. Commentators disagree about the translation of *yü* 竽 here—the character normally refers to a "reed pipe organ," which does not fit the context.

70. There is some disagreement among commentators about these characters (腥 臊 洒 酸 *xing sao sa suan*) and the specific smells indicated here.

71. This combination (疾養 *jiyang*) also occurs in *Xunzi* 4/45. It seems that most commentators emend *yang* 養 (nourish) to *yang* 癢 (itch). I translate it this way because the rest of the items distinguished by the form and body here (and in 4/45) consist of opposite terms. Moreover, *Xunzi* 9/5 presents *yang* as the opposite of this term for illness:

> 五疾上收而養之
> Those with the five illnesses should be raised up and collected in order to nourish them.
> (*Xunzi* 9/5)

72. The inclusion of speech and cause (or "reason") here is remarkable and difficult to explain. This character *shuo* 說 (translated as "speech" here) might also be read as *shui* "persuasion" or *yue* "pleasure." Neither option seems to make the line any easier to understand. "Pleasure" fits the pattern, but seems

redundant, and it does not, in any case, eliminate the problem of translating *gu* 故.

As it stands, the line suggests that speech and causes (persuasions and reasons?) are related to things like happiness and sadness. Moreover, this relation is in some way comparable to things like hot, cold, and fragrant smells.

73. The presence of the heartmind in the list of differentiating senses will be discussed in Chapter 3.

74. Paul Rakita Goldin makes the comparison between "distinguish" (*yi* 異) in this passage and Wittgenstein's "seeing as." I think this is useful. However, Goldin also worries about the incoherence of the view he attributes to the *Xunzi* passage, which, he fears, seems to present each sense as if it "apperceives" independently of the others. He concludes that the *Xunzi* "cannot mean" that the five senses apperceive separately, "but that the five senses, collectively apperceive reality." Unfortunately, the *Xunzi* passage says nothing about the five senses working collectively (although it does say that the heartmind depends on the senses in order to verify knowledge). Paul Rakita Goldin, *Rituals of the Way: The Philosophy of Xunzi* (Peru, Ill.: Open Court, 1999), 97.

75. This part of the passage does not mention objects at all. Moreover, the idea of differentiation evokes a system in which identity is constituted by contrasts, not by properties of objects.

76. Martin Heidegger, *Being and Time,* trans. J. Macquarrie and E. Robinson (Oxford: Basil Blackwell, 1962), 207.

77. This might be a case of what the *Zhengming* calls the senses' "recording their kinds, but not knowing."

78. See *Laozi* 14 and 35, cited in Chapter 2 footnote 12.

79. The term *zheng* 徵 may be translated as "verifying" or "summoning." Aside from mentioning the eyes and ears, the passage provides no other clue for how the heartmind goes about doing it. Discussions of knowledge frequently seem to involve tallying and measuring, thus "verifying" may be more appropriate here.

For reasons presented in Chapters 2 and 3, I suspect the process refers to something commonplace: the attempt to match things like what a person says with what he/she does.

80. I think form and sound are singled out here because they are the first items in the list of the things differentiated by the ears and eyes. Here they seem to function as a synecdoche for the kinds of aspects the ears and eyes differentiate.

81. It is possible to interpret eyes and ears here as standing in for all of the senses, but the prominent role of the eyes and ears in other descriptions of knowledge makes this less likely. For a full discussion of the role of seeing and hearing in knowledge, see Chapter 2.

82. Considering its awkwardness, it is also possible that this last line was originally an editorial comment that made its way into the text by mistake.

83. In his discussion of the *Zhengming* chapter of the *Xunzi*, A. S. Cua refers to chaotic "sense data," which, he says, are transformed by the mind into "evidential grounding for our knowledge." A. S. Cua, *Ethical Argumentation: A Study in Hsun Tzu's Moral Epistemology* (Honolulu: University of Hawaii Press, 1985), 31. Watson's translation of the passage cited above (*Xunzi* 22/19–21) also invokes sense data. "Because of this over-all

understanding, it [the mind] may rely upon the data of the ear and understand sounds correctly....But this over-all understanding must wait until it has received new data from the senses and matched it with the data already recorded in the mind concerning a particular class of objects, before it can arrive at a correct understanding of the objects." Watson, *Hsun Tzu,* 142–143.

Knoblock translates the section along the same lines, alluding to "sense impressions" as performing an evidential role in knowing. "Only when it rests on the evidence provided by the ear is it possible for this awareness of the defining characteristics to know sound...the mind's awareness of defining characteristics necessarily requires that the sense organ be impressed by the type of thing to which that sense organ [is sensitive]." Knoblock, *Xunzi,* 130.

84. Such a reading produces the following interpretation of this part of the passage. It seems to say that because there is verifying knowledge it is possible—by virtue of the eyes and ears—to have knowledge of form aspects and sounds aspects. In other words, verifying knowledge makes knowledge of form and sound aspects possible, which is perhaps a way of saying that verifying knowledge *is* knowledge of sound and form aspects in tandem. (Note that together "hear and see" [*wenjian* 聞 見] means "know" or "understand." See Chapter 2.) This verifying knowledge of form aspects and sound aspects appears to be undercut in some way by the fact that it "awaits" (depends upon?) some activity of the "heavenly officials" (a term that seems to include the heartmind itself because it too forms "intentional things" in *Xunzi* 22/16). This dependence seems to be restated in the next line in the form of one of the two requirements for the attribution of knowledge (i.e., the attribution of verifying knowledge?).

85. That is, there is a pragmatic feature to this kind of knowing that differentiates it from perception: the heartmind can verify sound aspects and form aspects, but unless it can articulate or explain things, no one will credit it with knowledge.

Chapter Two: Hearing and Seeing

1. See also *Xunzi* 21/62, page 20.

2. Again, the character *se* can be translated as "color" (as in "the five colors"), "face," or "sex." It is, in any case, visual. Here it seems to function as "looks," specifically those that are appealing, hence the translation. See below for an extended discussion of sounds and looks.

3. Yu is one of the legendary virtuous kings of Chinese prehistory.

4. See also *Mozi* 36/18 for a similar passage.

5. The passage is noteworthy for its strange claim that the noble person's heartmind is small. Some commentators emend the text for this reason, but that seems unnecessary, because their heartminds *are* relatively small in relation to the things that their way can achieve.

6. The characters I translate as "knowledge" (*zhi* 知) and "understanding" (*zhi* 智) seem quite close in use and appearance. *Xunzi* 22/5 explains them in terms of one another (see Chapter 1, footnote 54.) This explanation seems to say that the term "knowledge" applies to something located in people and the term "understanding" applies to knowledge that is in some sense unified with something.

7. This is an echo of the *Lunyu* 7/8, where the teacher holds up one corner and the student must be able to respond with the other three.

8. The reason for my translation of *er mu zhi shi* as "products of the ears and eyes" is provided in Chapter 4. The texts do not say what the ears and eyes produce, but my contention is that it is neither data nor reality.

9. In another version of this, the terms change slightly. Standards are "originated" by "checking" the *qing* (conditions? dispositions?) of the ears and eyes:

> 惡乎考之考先聖大王之事
> 惡乎原之
> 察眾之耳目之請
> 惡乎用之發而為政乎國察萬民而觀之
> How are they to be tested? They are to be tested on the deeds of the early sage kings. How are they to be originated? They are to be checked by the *qing* of the eyes and ears of the multitude. How are they to be applied? They are to be applied by being adopted in government and observing their effects on the masses.
> (*Mozi* 37/3–4)

10. I translate this *xun* as "accord." Graham seems to translate it as "through"—"If the channels inward through the eyes and ears are cleared." Graham, *Chuang-tzu: The Inner Chapters*, 69.

11. Perhaps the point is to contrast "according" with the channels to manipulating them in some way. Or perhaps the inward direction is a reversal of the normal outward direction of hearing and seeing.

12. On similar lines, the *Laozi* describes its *dao* via an inability to hear and see. Although the relevant passages also mention an inability to taste, use, and obtain it, they stress hearing and seeing slightly more. For example, see *Laozi* 35 (in the Conclusion). The other series speaks of *dao* in terms of a failure of seeing, hearing, and grasping.

> 視之而弗見名之曰微
> 聽之而弗聞命之曰希
> 抿之而弗得命之曰夷
> We look at it without seeing it;
> We name it, saying "minute."
> We listen to it, but without hearing it;
> We name it, saying "sparse."
> We grasp it, but do not obtain it;
> We name it, saying "level."
> (*Laozi* 14)

(The *ming* 名 in the first line is supplied from Text A.) These two examples confirm that the pairing of hearing and seeing extends to the *Laozi*, but the inclusion of taste, use, and grasping makes them less significant for this argument.

13. The passage reads,

> 將必不使老與遲者老與遲者
> 耳目不聰明股肱不畢強
> 聲不和調明不轉朴
> 將必使當年因其耳目之聰明
> 股肱之畢強聲之和調眉之轉朴
> [To strike the bells] one must not employ the aged or the young. Their ears and eyes are not keen and bright, their

> arms are not strong, their sound is not harmonious, and their [visual] expression does not change quickly.
> One must employ those in the prime of life, because of the keenness and clarity of their eyes and ears, the strength of their limbs, the harmony of their sound and the quick changes in their [visual] expression.
> (*Mozi* 32/21)

The terms I translate as "visual expression" are different in the two instances—the first is "clarity" and the second is "eyebrow." Because both refer to visual things, and seem to parallel the reference to sound, I do not translate them as referring to the bell's expression, but to the expression of the people themselves.

14. One *li* equals .415 kilometers.

15. The *Xunzi* argues in favor of focusing, noting that one can neither look at two things at once, nor hear two things at once:

> 行衢道者不至事兩君者不容
> 目不能兩視而明耳不能兩聽而聰
> One who walks both branches of a road does not arrive, one who serves two lords does not please them, the eye cannot look at two things with clarity, the ear cannot hear two things with keenness.
> (*Xunzi* 1/22)

16. The *Laozi* contains something that might count as another example, although it is not clear that desire is at issue. In its pronouncements about the nature of things, the *Laozi* seems to categorize the world in terms of squares, vessels, tones, and (visual) images (see *Laozi* 41 in the Conclusion).

17. In one particularly difficult to interpret case, the *Mencius* clearly distinguishes *sheng* 聲 (sound) from *yan* 言 (speech), saying *sheng* is the more powerful of the two. This might be variously understood as distinguishing speech from music, from reputation, or from tone. The line from the *Mencius* says,

> 仁言不如仁聲之入人深也
> Humane speech does not compare to humane *sheng* in how deeply it enters into a person.
> (*Mencius* 7A14)

18. The counterexamples that match speech with a different form of visual appearance are the *Lunyu* 1/3 and 12/20, cited above (see page 66).

19. The *Xunzi* also says,

> 聲無小而不聞
> 行無隱而不形
> No sound is so small that it is not heard,
> No action is so hidden that it does not have [visible] form.
> (*Xunzi* 1/25)

20. I leave the translation vague as to whether the petty person watches the noble person *while* he walks the way. That sense is not demanded by the original text, but it seems likely, since I take it that the way is not something that exists except insofar as it is enacted by someone.

21. This knowledge of speech and action does not apply to heaven, which, we are told, does not need to speak (*Lunyu* 17/19; *Mencius* 5A5).

22. According to the *Mozi*, the two are causally related:

言不信者行不果
If one's speech is not trustworthy, one's actions will have no results.
(*Mozi* 2/9)

23. The *Mozi* instructs its readers to emulate the district chief in matters of speech and action. The passage reads,

去若不善言
學鄉長之善言
去若不善行
學鄉長之善行
Dismiss what is not good to say, and learn what the head of the district considers good speech. Dismiss what is not good to do, and learn what the head of the district considers good action.
(*Mozi* 11/14–15)

24. The character discussed here is *xian* 賢, but my claim is about virtue in a general sense.

25. The passage refers to *Lunyu* 11/3, where "study of culture" is a third category for evaluation.

26. The passage is a restatement of *Lunyu* 11/3, where Zaiwo and Zigong are credited with good speaking skills (*yanyu* 言語), and the other three are credited with virtuous action (*dexing* 德行).

27. Perhaps for this reason, Yan Hui (*Lunyu* 11/14) chose not to speak much and the *Mozi* values wisdom over plenitude of speech (*Mozi* 2/13).

28. The *Xunzi* makes a similar claim. See *Xunzi* 27/50 in footnote 33.

29. The metaphor of speed in speech and action also appears in *Mozi* 2/12, which criticizes those who work at speech, while being slow to act (see page 79).

30. *Xunzi* 12/94–95 mentions that the eye sees only as far as the wall, while the ear hears as far as the village:

> 牆之外目不見也
> 里之前耳不聞也
> 而人主之守司遠者天下近者境內
> 不可不略知也....
> 耳目之明如是其狹也
> 人主之守司如是其廣也
> The eye does not see outside the compound walls. The ear does not hear beyond the village. Yet the ruler's guidance and governance cannot fail to have a general knowledge that goes as far as the world and as near as the boundaries of the state....The clarity of the ears and eyes is that narrow, the guidance and governance of the ruler is that immense.
> (*Xunzi* 12/94)

In reference to a filial person, *Xunzi* 27/87–88 describes speech as what persuades those in the *distance*, while movement or "action" ("walking," which it correlates with the eye) is what persuades/delights those who are *near*.

> 言為可聞所以說遠也
> 行為可見所以說近也

Because speech can be heard, therefore it delights the far. Because action can be seen, therefore it delights the near. (*Xunzi* 27/88)

Together these passages suggest that the sounds we hear (perhaps including hearsay) are not as easily confined as the shapes we see.

31. The passage appears in two versions:

言足以遷行者常之
不足以遷行者勿常
不足以遷行而常之是蕩口也
If there is speech that can modify action, take that as your constant. If it is not sufficient to modify action, then do not take it as your constant. If it is not sufficient to modify action and yet you take it as your constant, that is wasting your mouth.
(*Mozi* 47/18–19)

The other version changes the term "modify" to "repeat" and "initiate":

言足以復行者常之
不足以舉行者勿常
If there is speech that can be repeated in action, take that as your constant. If it is not sufficient to initiate action, then do not take it as your constant.
(*Mozi* 46/37–38)

32. The *Xunzi* passage is an exhortation to utilize worthy people:

夫言用賢者口也卻賢者行也口行相反

Saying that you will use the worthy is mouthing [words]. Rejecting the worthy is action. This is the mouth and the action opposing one another.
(*Xunzi* 14/14–15)

33. The passage reads,

口言善身行惡國妖之
治國者...除其妖
When people's mouths speaks of good, but their bodies act badly, the state demonizes them. Those who govern the state...cast off its demons.
(*Xunzi* 27/50–51)

34. There may be some ambiguity as to whether this means looking inside through the pupil or looking at the pupil itself. However, because the issue is the pupil's brightness or dullness, this seems to be a case of looking *at* the pupil, where the interior of the person manifests itself.

Chapter Three: The Heartmind's Relation to the Senses

1. I focus on pondering here because, although the heartmind is said to "think" as well as "ponder," "pondering" is its more well-described function.

2. Again, the term *qing* is ambiguous, hence the translation. (See Chapter 1, footnote 59.)

3. The *Zhuangzi* also mentions self-selecting as part of the image of how heaven motivates movement. When asked about something called the "pipes of heaven," a character replies:

夫吹萬不同而使其自已也

> 咸其自取怒者其誰邪
> Who is it who impels things by puffing out the ten thousand differences, by controlling their self-ending, and stimulating their self-selecting?
> (*Zhuangzi* 2/8–9)

The *Xunzi* also refers to an instance where the heartmind picks people (for office):

> 以其可道之心取人
> 則合於道人
> If you select people by using the [kind of] heartmind that affirms the way, then you will unite with people of the way.
> (*Xunzi* 21/33)

Even this inconsequential looking selection for office seems worth noting, because it belongs to this pattern of the heartmind selecting.

4. In order to make sense of the line, "pupil" here is traditionally taken to mean "look down," "scrutinize," or "stare at."

5. As I argue elsewhere, Graham's reconstruction seems to depend crucially upon an unconvincing scheme that he created to explain the structure of the Canons. It is possible that some of his translations are reliable, but the reconstruction as a whole depends upon a faulty foundation. Thus, any individual piece of it should be used with caution and be subject to critical reassessment. See my "Critique of A. C. Graham's Reconstruction of the Neo-Mohist Canons," *Journal of the American Oriental Society* 119 (1): 1–11.

The passage cited here is from A. C. Graham, *Later Mohist Logic, Ethics and Science* (Hong Kong: Chinese University Press, 1978).

6. The line reads,

瞽者仰視而不見星
The blind person looks up, but does not see the stars.
(*Xunzi* 21/72–73)

7. It is not clear what the heartmind "obtains." However, both Canon A4 and *Mencius* 6A15 refer to "obtaining it." The metaphor comparing what the heartmind obtains to a needle seems to preclude interpreting "obtain" as something abstract, as in saying the heartmind "realizes" or "achieves."

If pondering itself is the selection of *qing* (as *Xunzi* 22/3 suggests), and pondering is different from knowing (as *Xunzi* 24/2 suggests), then knowing must be something other than just selecting *qing*. Perhaps it is the "arrival" at *qing* referred to in *Xunzi* 21/47.

8. See also *Mencius* 1A7 and *Mozi* 16/54–55.

9. For example, *Mencius* 5B1.

10. The inclusion of speech within a list of things distinguished by the senses may not be as unusual as it seems. As Constance Classen points out, the Christian interpreter Philo considered speech to be one of the five senses. Classen, *Worlds of Sense*, 2.

11. See pages 44–45 for another discussion of this passage.

12. See page 48 for a fuller citation of this passage.

13. There is a close connection between *ming* 命 and *ming* 名. The initial reference to the process uses the character *ming* 命 (*ran hou sui er ming zhi* 然後隨而命之, "Thereupon, follow and decree names for them"), but, as the *Xunzi* begins to elaborate on the details of how *ming* 命 should work, it is clearly a matter of applying names (*ming* 名). *Xunzi* 22/21–25.

14. After describing the heartmind as empty, in spite of its storage of aims, the passage says that knowledge requires sameness and difference:

> 心生而有知知而有異異也者同時兼知之
> 同時兼知之兩也
> 然而有所謂一
> 不以夫一害此一謂之壹
> Once the heartmind is born, there is knowledge, once there is knowledge, there are differences. Differences are collectively known at one time. Things collectively known at one time are multiple [lit. "two"]. And yet it has what can be called unity. Not letting "that one" damage "this one" is called "unity."

The passage ends with a comment about dreaming:

> 心臥則夢偷則自行使之則謀故心未嘗不動也
> 然而有所謂靜
> 不以夢劇亂知謂之靜
> When the heartmind sleeps, it dreams. When it is not occupied, then it goes off on its own. When it is put to use, then it plans. Therefore, the heartmind never stops moving, and yet it has what can be called calmness. Not allowing dreams and disturbances to disorder knowledge is called "calmness."
> (*Xunzi* 21/38–39)

15. The *Mozi* says,

其心不察其智而與其愛
The heartminds of [the rulers] share their favor [with certain people] without examining their understanding.
(*Mozi* 9/37)

16. Lao Kan, "The Early Use of the Tally in China," in *Ancient China: Studies in Early Civilization,* ed. David T. Roy and Tsuen-hsuin Tsien (Hong Kong: Chinese University Press, 1978). This ancient conception seems to carry over to the present day in China with the expression for asking whether something is correct: 對不對 [lit. "Does it match or not match?"].

17. The passage reads,

心有徵知
徵知則
緣耳而知聲可也
緣目而知形可也
There is verifying knowledge; thus, because of [lit. caused by] the ear, it is possible to know sounds; because of [caused by] the eye, it is possible to know forms.
(*Xunzi* 22/19)

18. The passage says,

心者形之君也
The heartmind is the ruler of the form.
(*Xunzi* 21/44)

19. The term *tian* 天 here contrasts to human. See Chapter 1, note 14.

20. Watson's translation makes no sense of the *shi* 使, so it substitutes a *bi* 蔽 instead, making the last line read "How much more so with a man whose mind is obsessed!" Watson, *Hsun Tzu*, 122.

21. *Xunzi* 22/19.

22. Two passages from the *Xunzi* note that the senses cannot substitute for one another: *Xunzi* 17/11 and *Xunzi* 12/61 (see page 19).

23. In other cases, like the *Zhengming* and *Xunzi* 10/61–63, the passage lists the heartmind along with the senses, but distinguishes it as well. (*Xunzi* 10/63 uses a different term preceding the heartmind from the term it uses for the other senses.)

24. Again, I am translating the *Mawangdui* edition of the *Laozi* here, unless otherwise noted, but for the readers' convenience, I am using the more familiar *Wang Bi* chapter numbers.

The order of the items in the *Wang Bi* edition places the heartmind last.

25. The *Mozi* contains a list of what could be senses, but the subject of the passage is not desire. Even if it is not a sense list, it is noteworthy that, once again in relation to the person as a whole, the heartmind's place is not necessarily at the high point of the list (see *Mozi* 12/65–67, page 26).

26. *Xunzi* 22/20.

27. In other words, vision and hearing operate best at close range.

28. See discussion of wind in Chapter 1.

29. It does not store represented images or sense data.

30. The passage says,

人心譬如槃水正錯而勿動
則湛濁在下而清明在上
則足以見鬒眉而察理矣
微風過之湛濁動乎下清明亂於上
則不可以得大形之正也
The human heartmind is like a pan of water. If you place the pan upright and do not move it, then heavy muddiness will be at the bottom and clear brightness will be at the top. Then it will be sufficient to see the hair and eyebrows and examine the [facial] lines. [But if] a slight wind passes it, then the heavy muddiness moves on the bottom, and the clear brightness is disordered on the top. Then you cannot even obtain [from it] a large form's alignment.
(*Xunzi* 21/55–56)

It is noteworthy that wind is what disturbs the heartmind's operations. The person is like water in this regard: wind is a potent cause of transformation, both positive and negative. (See the discussion in Chapter 1 where *de* fills the person like a body of water.)

31. Another way to read the passage is to take the first line as "Strange forms and alienated heartminds." I translate it this way because the *jiao* 交 in the next line is the same term used in *Mencius* 6A15 to describe the operations of the senses in relation to things.

32. It is not clear how exactly this peace manages to be emitted, but the same verb is used to describe how speech exits from the mouth in both the *Lunyu* 4/22 and *Xunzi* 20/26.

33. I take this first line as a reference to "rectifying" one's actual physical body, hence I read the "enter" as being like the strange sense of "entering someone's enclosure [body?]" in *Zhuangzi* 4/29. This translation is ambiguous, but it resembles the original that is also not so clear about what would enter what when the form approaches. Watson does not take the *zheng ru shen* as concretely referring to rectifying one's physical body. He translates it as "make sure you yourself are in the right" (Watson, *Chuang Tzu*, 62). This allows him to take the thing approached to be the other person's behavior and translate *ru* 入 as "pulled in with him." Graham's translation of the first line could be taken to refer to the physical body: "Get your own person rightly adjusted!" but he too translates *jiu* as "get close" and *ru* as "drawn in" without indicating to *what* (Graham, *Chuang-tzu*, 72).

Chapter Four: Names and Their "Filling"

1. The *Zhuangzi* indicates that "names and *shi*" demarcate a fundamental division. *Zhuangzi* 7/23–24 tells a story of a teacher making fun of the practice of reading physiognomy. The teacher performs a process that seems like regression, in which he "shows" himself to the physiognomist at certain primal states. Along the way, he reaches a very basic state wherein "names and *shi* have not entered, but impulses come up from his heels" (名實不入而機發於踵).

2. The glosses in the *Shuo wen* are not presented as definitions (i.e., the essence of a term, in the form of its meanings). Rather, the glosses are lists of how the character is

used, from which one may infer its meanings (in the sense of how the character functions within the language of the texts).

3. In the *Mencius*, *shi* appears twice in conjunction with *chong* 充 (fill). *Mencius* 7B25 and 7B31.

4. For example, this use appears in *Laozi* 3.

5. See J. L. Austin's *Sense and Sensibilia* for an analysis of the many ways we employ the term "reality." J. L. Austin, *Sense and Sensibilia* (New York: Oxford University Press, 1962).

6. Although *shi* is contrasted to a variety of things, only emptiness can truly be considered its opposite, in the sense that a thing cannot be simultaneously empty and *shi*.

Other terms contrast to *shi* without quite being opposites. Names are often the pair term for *shi*—a relation that is more parallel than oppositional (as I will argue below). The *Xunzi* contains a case of *shi* being juxtaposed to *ci* 辭 (phrases). The *Xunzi* 22/39 explains the character *ci* 辭 as "an amalgam of names for different *shi*, laying out one intent.":

> 惠子蔽於辭而不知實....
> 由辭謂之道盡論矣
> Huizi is clouded by phrases and does not know *shi* [fruition? fulfillment?]....
> If you address things by starting from phrases [lit. "if your 'call' on things starts from phrases"], then the way will be entirely about sorting.
> (*Xunzi* 21/22–26)

The *Zhuangzi* refers to a similar kind of relation in a passage juxtaposing *shi* to *wen* 文. Using a sexual metaphor, the *Zhuangzi* implies that the fruit is like the male half of a pair, which is required to fill out the form, so that something can be born:

> 吾與汝既其文未既其實
> 而固得道與
> 眾雌而無雄而又奚卵焉
> With you I have exhausted the form, but not yet exhausted the fruits: how could you have a sure grasp of the way? With so many hens but no cock, what eggs can you expect from them?
> (*Zhuangzi* 7/18)

7. In the *Mozi*, *qing* and *shi* are interchanged in reference to reliable conditions, as well as in reference to ears and eyes (for the latter, see Chapter 2). The *Mozi* indicates something worthy of trust via "fullness" (*shi*) and being rooted in "conditions/dispositions" (*qing*):

> 今天下之王公大人士君子請將欲富其國家...
> Now, if the rulers and the gentlemen of the world *qing* [by condition/disposition?] desire to enrich their country...
> (*Mozi* 12/74–75)

> 今天下之士君子忠實欲天下之富...
> Now, if the gentlemen of the world sincerely and *shi* [fully] desire to have the world be rich...
> (*Mozi* 35/46)

The sincerity that is connected to these terms may relate to being in alignment with the center of the heartmind (or, the center that *is* the heartmind). The use of *zhong* 忠 in the first example switches with *zhong* 中 "central" in other passages (assuming that we should sooner translate *zhong* as "central" than "inside" in the context of heaven). For example,

> 若天之中實不愛此民也
> **If heaven did not centrally and *shi* [fully] love the people...**
> *Mozi* 28/25

However (apropos of the discussion of authenticity and emotions below), even if *qing* is interpreted as "dispositions" or "feelings," this is not to say that sincere emotions are private entities located inside a center (the heartmind) and not manifest on the outside. Sincere authenticity need not derive from being located inside the heartmind, but simply from being aligned with its centrality.

It is worth noting that, although *qing* 情 and *shi* 實 seem interchangeable in such contexts, their use still implies something slightly different. *Qing* seems to refer to what is present particularly from birth (*Xunzi* 23/26), whereas *shi* seems to indicate a fulfilled product. This point was clarified for me by Chris Fraser (personal communication).

8. The following evidence is the basis for my characterization of heaven and earth: *Zhuangzi* 4/88 notes that earth is heavy. In a story in *Zhuangzi*, Huzi contrasts earth to heaven in a way that suggests the earth is damp and cold, whereas heaven is hot and bright (*Zhuangzi* 7/21 and 7/23). When it rains, heaven can become *yin* 陰, but this is not its usual state (*Mencius* 2A4). Heaven is described as bright (*Zhuangzi* 2/29; *Xunzi* 20/29; and *Mozi* 48/50, although the reference is to its intelligence). Heaven is associated with the sun and/or the moon or light and darkness in *Xunzi* 17/40, *Mencius* 5A4, and *Zhuangzi* 6/21.

The question of superiority is only a matter of degree, because heaven and earth form a continuum, but heaven usually seems the more imposing of the two.

9. As Norbert Elias points out, there is some confusion in the way we speak of emotions. We speak of them both in a broad sense—as having somatic, behavioral, and feeling components—and in a narrow sense, as if they were only the feeling component. The latter is implied when we speak of "expressing emotions," which Elias notes "is representative of a human self-image according to which the true self of a person is hidden deep inside—one cannot quite be sure inside of what." According to Elias, this "common sense" concept of emotion reflects an inadequate image of human beings. Norbert Elias, "On Human Beings and Their Emotions: A Process-Sociological Essay," in *Theory, Culture, & Society* 4: 355–356.

We should be cautious lest that common-sense concept of emotion not be shared by early Chinese texts. *Zhuangzi* 3/18 mentions that one should not let sadness and happiness enter:

> 安時而處順哀樂不能入也
> If one is content with the times and following on the course, sadness and joy cannot enter.
> (*Zhuangzi* 3/18)

This "entering" makes no sense if one takes emotions to be private entities/events. However, if emotions include their public expression, the passage could refer to protecting oneself from being affected by the (expressed and manifest) emotions of others.

For an argument against the existence of inaccessible psychological states in the *Lunyu*, see Herbert Fingarette, *Confucius—The Secular as Sacred* (New York: Harper and Row, 1972), 37–56. See also Mary Bockover's argument that "the line between internal and external feelings is...arbitrary," as well as her use of Robert Solomon's claims that emotions are like actions, insofar as they are intentional or "about something." Mary I. Bockover, "The Concept of Emotion Revisited: A Critical

Synthesis of Western and Confucian Thought," in *Emotions in Asian Thought: A Dialogue in Comparative Philosophy*, 163.

10. An alternate translation, even more favorable to my reading, takes *dui* 兑 as *yue* 悦 and reads the line as "make it so that harmony and ease circulate, but there is no loss in joy."

11. The reader may be reminded of the Warring States understanding of health as dynamic movement, referred to in the Introduction.

12. The passage chastises Hui Shi for letting something like emotions (likes and dislikes) harm him on the inside. Contrasting Hui Shi to sages, the character Zhuangzi says,

> 道與之貌天與之形無以好惡內傷其身
> 今子外乎子之神勞乎子之精
> 倚樹而吟據槁梧而瞑
> 天選子之形子以堅白鳴
> The way gives such people their manner, heaven gives them their shape.
> They do not use likes and dislikes to inwardly wound their bodies.
> Now you, sir, keep on externalizing your *shen* [spirits] and overworking your *jing* [seminal powers], with your intoning, while you lean on a tree, and dozing, while you lean on your study desk.
> Heaven selected your shape, but you use "hard" and "white" to chirp.
> (*Zhuangzi* 5/58–60)

13. Instead of testing against the five senses, there are occasional instances of something like "seeing for oneself"—perhaps because the eye sees what is near and close in time. Most

often, the eyes, ears, and heartmind play the verifying role that one might expect to be played collectively by all of the senses. It is true that when the *Xunzi* explains how the five senses function, it mentions that verifying knowledge depends on the heavenly officers fitting their kinds. However, the *Xunzi* seems to think only the heartmind's dependence on the eyes and ears merits elaboration (*Xunzi* 22/19–20). (For more discussion of this topic, see Chapter 3)

14. The passage then points out the "beauty" of names, which could refer to their visual aspect, but the term *wen* 文 can also be applied to speech, and hence is not necessarily visual:

> 名聞而實喻名之用也
> 累而成文名之麗也
> 用麗俱得謂之知名
> When a name is heard and a *shi* is understood, that is the function of names.
> When names are bound and become ornate, that is the beauty of names.
> Obtaining both the use and the beauty of names, [we] call this "knowing names."
> (*Xunzi* 22/38)

15. For the connection between *ming* 名 and *ming* 命, see Marcel Granet, *La Penseé Chinoise* (Paris: Albin Michel, 1968), 366, and Graham, *Later Mohist Logic, Ethics and Science*, 199.

16. This is an example of a translation by Graham, with its characteristic emendations based on his proposed structure for the Canons. The reader should be warned that the translation involves emending three characters (indicated by the asterisks). The translation of *bi* 必 (must) as "necessarily requires" reflects

Graham's (to my mind erroneous) view that this portion of the Canons belongs to the realm of necessary, atemporal logic.

It is not clear to me what name Graham means by "the name" in the last line.

17. William Boltz writes that from 500 B.C.E. on—until *zi* 字 replaced it—"the term *ming* 名 is used meaning 'word' of either the spoken or written language of equal force." William Boltz, *The Origin and Early Development of the Chinese Writing System* (New Haven: American Oriental Society, 1994), 138. Although I am not sure I understand what Boltz means by "of equal force," I suspect my argument disagrees with his claim, that is, my impression is that *ming* rarely refers to writing in these texts, and if it occasionally does, the writing of *ming* implicitly refers to a record of sounds, because *ming* is predominantly oral/aural.

Boltz's own argument is concerned with the actual history of writing (rather than the early Chinese perception of it). Still, as a whole, Boltz's argument highlights the oral/aural aspects of *ming*. Boltz notes that the character *ming* 名, in its origin, is a picture of a mouth, to which the 夕 graph (which, he argues, is pronounced *ming* in this case) is added to specify the pronunciation. See *The Origin and Early Development of the Chinese Writing System,* 105. He himself hints that the sense of *ming* as writing is an extension of its aural/oral sense. He argues that the graph *ming* 銘 developed later than *ming* 名 as an attempt to specify an *inscribed* name. Thus, his argument suggests that the character *ming* 銘 does not testify to the visuality of *ming* 名. On the contrary, it implies that *ming* 名 referred to sounds, while *ming* 銘 referred to inscribed sounds. See *The Origin and Early Development of the Chinese Writing System*, 70.

18. I do not understand why Graham translates *qi ming* as "making a name for yourself." His translation reads,

> I shall tell you. You are capable of entering and roaming free inside his cage, but do not be excited that you are making a name for yourself. When the words penetrate, sing your native note; when they fail to penetrate, desist. (*Zhuangzi* 4/29; Graham, *Chuang-tzu*, 69)

19. Because of the pattern of the texts using expressions like "hear without listening" and "see without looking," the reference to "naming without seeing" in the *Laozi* 47 might appear to indicate a visual aspect of naming. However, the line prior to "naming without seeing" reads "knows without going," rather than "knows without thinking/pondering." Thus, the completed actions in that chapter do not have the kind of automatic cause-effect relation that would establish seeing as the ordinary causal prelude to naming.

20. The *Xunzi* contains an example of the former type:

> 欲養其名而亂其行
> [Certain people] want to nourish their names [fame], but instead they disorder their actions.
> (*Xunzi* 22/83)

21. In other instances where *shi* is the pair term for speech, both "reality" and "action" may seem like equally plausible translations. For instance, *shi* functions as a pair term for speech (*yan*) in the *Zhuangzi* 5/49. The *Zhuangzi* relates a story of a ruler saying this to "Confucius":

> 始也吾以南面而君天下
> 執民之紀而憂其死吾自以為至通矣
> 今吾聞至人之言恐吾無其實
> 輕用吾身而亡其國

> Earlier, I thought I had ultimate understanding of facing south, being lord of the world, controlling the regulation of the people, and worrying about their deaths.
> Now I have heard the speech of an "ultimate-person." I fear I lack your [or "its"] *shi*, have lightly treated my person, and will lose my country.
> (*Zhuangzi* 5/48–49)

While "reality" is a possible translation, the use of *shi* as the pair term for speech argues for translating *shi* as a form of action. On such a reading, the king hears Confucius's speech and realizes that his prior acts of controlling and worrying have not been in accord with it. On my reading, rather than lacking the reality or substance referred to by Confucius's speech, the king lacks the actions that correspond to it.

22. Compare Lau's translation:

> Words without reality are ill-omened, and the reality of the ill-omened will befall those who stand in the way of good people.
> (*Mencius* 4B17; Lau, *Mencius*, 130)

There is no *zhe* 者 to justify supplying a "the" before "ill-omened." Technically, if the *shi* is "reality," then it should read "the reality of being ill-omened."

As I argue below, the greater disseminating power of speech perhaps accounts for why the *Mencius* refers to *yan* without *shi* as inauspicious, without saying that *shi* without *yan* is inauspicious.

23. See *Zhuangzi* 4/49–50 (page 73).

24. While it does not pair *shi* with *yan*, a passage from the *Zhengming* is equally well served by interpreting *shi* as an act of fulfillment, rather than reality:

> 名無固宜約之以命
> 約定俗成謂之宜
> 異於約則謂之不宜
> 名無固實約之以命實
> 約定俗成謂之實名
>
> Names have no original appropriateness. Bind them by decree/ordaining. When the binding settles and a habit forms, call it appropriate.
> If it is different from the habit, then call it inappropriate.
> Names have no original *shi* [fulfillment?]. Bind them by ordaining *shi*. If the binding settles and a habit forms, call it a *shi* name [a full name? a fruitful name?].
> (*Xunzi* 22/25–27)

For those who interpret *shi* as "real," this passage seems to say that names have no original reality. Sticking to the grammatical pattern, the second claim sounds like a rephrasing of the first ("names have merely conventional appropriateness" and "names have merely conventional reality"). But this redundancy seems out of place, because the next line is not at all redundant. Instead of saying that names have merely conventional goodness, it asserts that names have original goodness, which gives the impression that the passage is not simply repeating the same thing in different forms.

Translating *shi* in terms of an act that brings something to fruition helps resolve the problem. By such a reading, after noting that names have merely conventional appropriateness, the passage adds that names have no original filling. In other words, not only is the appropriateness of names themselves conventional (i.e., what *sounds* count as names), but the fulfillment of names (i.e., what *actions/events* count as filling a name) is also conventional.

25. Although a significant amount of the evidence for this part of the argument derives from the *Mozi*, that does not, I think, argue for restricting its conclusions to the *Mozi*. Unless there is explicit evidence to the contrary, it seems safe to assume that ideas about the sensory nature of fundamental categories of experience—such as the notion that *ming/shi* is an aural/visual pair—are not likely to belong to isolated texts.

26. Discriminating the *wu* is the visual counterpart to using the names. The *qi* 其 before *wu* 物 refers back to *ming* in the prior line.

27. Breaking up the line differently points to an alternate reading: "They are not able [to pick]. It is a matter of knowledge."

28. It is interesting to note that some scholars argue that, during the Shang dynasty, *wu* 物 was originally a color term, as well as a term used to mean "to select on the basis of color." Wang Tao, "Color Terms in Shang Oracle Bone Inscriptions," *Bulletin of the School of Oriental and African Studies* 59: 82.

29. This line is part of the corrupted chapters known as the Neo-Mohist Canons. While the line I cite involves no changing of the text, Graham's reconstruction of the passage as a whole is emended in places:

A 80 知 * 聞 說 親 名 實 合 為
（知）傳 受 之 聞 也 方 不 * 運 說 也
身 觀 焉 親 也 所 以 謂 名也 所 謂 實 也
名 實 耦 合 也 志 行 為 也

> C. *Chih* (know). By hearsay, by explanation, by personal experience. The name, the object, how to relate, how to act.
> E. Having received it at second hand is knowing by 'hearsay.' Knowing that something square will not rotate is by 'explanation.' Having been a witness oneself is knowing 'by personal experience.'
> What something is called by is its 'name.' What is so called is the 'object.' The mating of name and object is 'relating.' To intend and to perform are 'to act.'
> (Graham, *Later Mohist Logic Ethics and Science*, 327)

Note that the three uses of "by" in the first line are not indicated in any way in the Chinese. The reader should also be aware that the two asterisks represent two emendations. The second emendation that produces "something square will not rotate" seems particularly unconvincing. Graham thinks that the Canons contain four main sections, one of which is "necessary knowledge" or logic. Given that knowledge is the topic of the Canon, he may have felt obliged, or at least encouraged, to locate some kind of logical necessity in this Canon. Thus, this phrase attached to *shuo* 說 (speech/spoken explanation)—which contains an unidentifiable character—is manipulated to sound like logic.

30. The topic of each Canon is supposed to be indicated by the first word.

31. See Fingarette's discussion of performative language and the rectification of names (Fingarette, *Confucius—Secular as Sacred*, 15). For the theory of rectifying names in the *Lunyu* in light of a prescriptive view of language, see Hansen, *Daoist Theory of Chinese Thought*, 65–71. See also Carine Defoort's categorization of various interpretations of rectification of names in the *Lunyu*. Carine Defoort, *The Pheasant Cap Master: A*

Rhetorical Reading (Albany: State University of New York Press, 1997), 168–177.

32. The rectification of names passage in the *Lunyu* (13/3, cited below) does not mention *shi*.

33. It also calls it "chaotic" (*Xunzi* 22/11).

34. Even with the alternate reading, "names are the reason that *shi* are met and bound," the element that needs binding still seems to be the *shi*.

35. Given other *Zhuangzi* passages that imply that the heartmind dies (2/20) or that a living person cannot know whether the heartmind dies (2/80–85), Confucius's claim here that the heartmind never dies may be an indication of his less-than-complete understanding (assuming that there is consistency in the viewpoint in the *Zhuangzi* in this regard). In any case, whether or not the passage reflects the position of the authors of the *Zhuangzi*, Confucius supplies what he supposes to be an easily recognizable example. Thus, the priorities reflected in his example appear to be commonplace.

36. The earlier lines of this passage say that names are bound. Now this line says that ordaining binds *shi*. This implies that there is a difference between binding names to *shi* and just binding names. My guess is that "binding names" refers to binding sounds to one another, which will thenceforth count as names.

37. This last claim comes as a surprise—what is the difference between appropriateness and goodness, such that names lack original appropriateness yet possess original goodness? The passage does not elaborate on the nature of "appropriateness." It explains "goodness" as directness and ease, as well as absence of

contrariness. However, these things seem as descriptive of appropriateness as they are of goodness.

Interpreting the entire passage in terms of writing rather than sounds in no way alleviates the confusion. Whether one "binds" sounds or elements of written characters, the passage still fails to address why something that is good, easy, and not contrary should not be called "originally appropriate" if it is going to be called "originally good."

Perhaps the reason names have *original* goodness is that some things, like simplicity, always help in naming, regardless of whether habit succeeds in making the name appropriate.

38. Graham's translation is extremely suspicious in this regard. For the second question, he substitutes *shi* for "guest," and translates it so that it reads, "Would it be for the sake of the substance?" (Graham, *Chuang-tsu*, 45). His translation implies that the second motivation would be more appealing than the first. In this way, he alters the tone of the passage entirely, making it sound like a critique of names as "mere" guests of substances.

39. In *Mozi* 28/39 and *Xunzi* 22/1, names are "appended." In *Xunzi* 22/2, names are "located in."

40. The *Xunzi* describes this as the condition under the reign of good rulers:

> 名定而實辨
> Names are settled, and thereupon *shi* are distinguished.
> (*Xunzi* 22/7)

41. This is probably a reference to Yan Hui.

42. Just as names have the potential to be empty, so too speech has the potential to be flowery. The *Xunzi* associates speech with flowers, also contrasting speech to action:

> 奮於言者華
> 奮於行者伐色
> A person who disperses his/her speech is flowery.
> A person who disperses his/her actions is showing off.
> (*Xunzi* 29/26)

For more on plant metaphors in early China, see Donald Munro's "The Family Network, the Stream of Water, and the Plant" in *Individualism and Holism: Studies in Confucian and Taoism Values*, 259–292.

43. Lau and Ames translation modified. D. C. Lau and Roger T. Ames, trans., *Yuan Dao: Tracing Dao to Its Source* (New York: Ballatine Books, 1998), 80.

44. The passage simply says that names "hang," but another passage from the *Xunzi* constructs an analogy between names and measurement standards, which argues for this reading. The *Xunzi* says,

> 故析辭擅作名
> 以亂正名
> 使民疑惑
> 人多辨訟
> 則謂之大姦
> 其罪猶為符節度量之罪也
> 故其民莫敢託為奇辭以亂正名
> To be sure, those who split phrases and, on their own authority, create names in order to disorder correct names, make people suspicious and confused and increase people's

> debates and disputes. Hence, this is called great treachery, and their crime is [treated] like those who violate tallies or weights and measures.
> Hence, [the true ruler's] people do not dare to make up strange phrases and disorder correct names.
> (*Xunzi* 22/7–9)

An individual who threatens the orderly relation of names to *shi*, is like someone who tampers with weights and measures, hence the metaphor of names "hanging" might be that of a standard of measure.

45. However, spoken names presumably would not penetrate as deeply as music, because, according to one interpretation, *Mencius* 7A14 seems to say that "tone" is much more effective than the speech itself (see Chapter 2 note 17).

Chapter Five: Conclusion

1. Like Knoblock, I take *xing* 形 to be 型 "instructions." Knoblock, *Xunzi*, 2:19.

2. According to Kenneth DeWoskin, in early Chinese music theory, music functions by mutual resonance rather than one side being the cause and the other exhibiting the effect. Describing how music functions in the *Book of Music*, DeWoskin writes,

> The 'Book of Music' defines a process that is closer to sympathetic resonance than to causation. Confounding attempts at definitive translation, the verb *kan* 感 means, on the one hand, to 'impinge,' 'affect,' or 'move' and, on the other hand, 'perceive,' 'feel,' or 'sense';...the 'Book of Music' notes the significant concurrence of 'coarse sound'

and a 'mind moved to anger' without attempting to establish the agency, or causality, of the concurrence.

Kenneth DeWoskin, *A Song for One or Two: Music and the Concept of Art in Early China* (Ann Arbor, Mich.: Center for Chinese Studies, The University of Michigan, 1982), 97.

3. Interestingly, the *Xunzi* does not always describe the road as straight, although usually it does.

4. When *Xunzi* expresses its concern about resonating with inappropriate desires, it calls it "complying" with the desire of the ears and eyes, rather than "responding" to them, but it does not explain the difference (see *Xunzi* 23/2, page 51).

5. The *Xunzi* describes the response as inexhaustible:

應變不窮
是聖人之辯者也
Responding to changes without limit:
Such is the discussion of the sage.
(*Xunzi* 5/60)

6. The phrasing here is reminiscent of *wuwei* 無為, and it particularly resembles the way it is applied to sensory contexts in the *Laozi*.

7. The term I translate as "well-spoken" here is *bian* 辯 (discuss, debate). The comparison with the senses suggests that oral discussion simply is what the scholar does, just as the eye sees.

The phrase *lou zhi* 僂指 "bend a finger" is not clear.

8. In this case, the character *qu* 曲, which most often appears in contrast to *zheng* 正 "straight," hence meaning

"divergent" or "crooked," may be better read as "sprouts" or "small things."

9. Aside from implying that too much effort of the eyes and ears is impractical, the *Xunzi* also criticizes the unseen and unheard because, by not providing anything auditory and visual, they make resonance impossible (as in 18/1 [above], where the *Xunzi* compares the ruler to a singing master).

10. Again, what I am translating as "acting" is a character that also means "walk," "go," or "proceed." That "acting" is connected with "walking" has to be important in a context where the ultimate goal is to follow the proper *dao,* "way" or "path."

11. A similar passage in the *Shuo Yuan* has slightly different elements. Knoblock notes that in the *Shuo Yuan* version, the hand is best. "The ear's hearing something is not as good as the eye's seeing it; the eye's seeing it is not as good as the foot's treading upon it; the foot's treading on it is not as good as the hand's differentiating it" (Knoblock, *Xunzi,* 2:289).

12. Perhaps the closeness of seeing might refer to the sense of being able to "see for oneself." The *Xunzi* never mentions "seeing for oneself" as a particular asset of visual sensation, but the *Mencius* does (*Mencius* 1B8). On the other hand, perhaps this is not something that the *Xunzi* views as exclusive to the visual modality—it is also possible to hear for oneself.

13. The emphasis on body here suggests the embodied person and should not be seen in terms of a contrast to the heartmind.

14. The translation of *gu* in this context is difficult. In other contexts, it functions as 'reason,' 'cause,' 'formerly,' and 'to die.'

15. The *Xunzi* often describes the aim of knowing in pragmatic terms. It does not speak of knowing as being correct for its own sake, but speaks instead of resolving doubts (*Xunzi* 12/104), responding to ten thousand changes (*Xunzi* 12/103), and avoiding the misfortune of the heartmind's aims not being clear (*Xunzi* 22/53). According to the *Xunzi*, the ancients examined knowledge and thinking on the basis of their completion, just as they measured action and repose on the basis of ritual (*Xunzi* 12/74).

16. Having said that speech need not aim to rectify action, *Mencius* 7B37 still criticizes people whose speech and action do not take note of each other (presumably in order to rectify one another). In fact, in *Mencius* 3B9 (see page 106), Mencius is said to view his own speech as aimed at stopping the heterodox speech and action of other thinkers.

17. This might be read as simply ranking trust and productivity below doing what is right, but such a reading requires ignoring the specific terminology—*bu bi xin* here and *bi xin* in 7B33.

18. The implicit contrast to "broad" learning argues for translating this *yue* as "concise," rather than "bound" as in the *Zhengming*.

19. This metaphor of *bu xia dai*, which I translate as "below the belt," is rendered "below the girdle" by Legge *(The Works of Mencius*, 495) and "below the sash" by Lau (*Mencius*, 201). I do not know whether the same connotations as "below the belt" apply here.

20. When it does appear, it refers to a response to a question (*Mencius* 2B8, 2B11, and 6B1).

21. This extension from center to periphery suggests that the emotion is not entirely subjective and intrapersonal. Thus, when the *Mencius* 6A4–5 debates whether humaneness and rightness are internal or external, being internal does not seem to mean completely private. It is more like beginning internally.

22. As Kwong-loi Shun notes, "...Mencius probably regarded the physical form as having some kind of ethical dimension...one's ethical qualities are inevitably manifested in one's physical form—it is because they are so manifested that they can be discerned by others and can have a transformative effect." Kwong-loi Shun, *Mencius and Early Chinese Thought* (Stanford: Stanford University Press, 1997), 162–163.

23. In this case, the origin of the similarity is the person's position, rather than the heartmind; however, the principle is the same, insofar as the origin functions as cause.

Another possible reading of the passage is that the princes' accents sound alike because they grew up in the same area. However, this reading seems to make the *Mencius*'s point needlessly banal.

24. See *Mencius* 4A16 (page 82). Because the issue is the pupil's brightness or dullness, this seems to be a case of the central part of the person manifesting itself in the pupil, rather than a matter of looking inside a person through their pupils.

25. The *Mencius* considers only one instance of a duplicitous person, who says that he will do something but does not follow through. The *Mencius* does not seem to see any particular

problem in this. The advisors of the prince in question simply recognize the situation and depart (see *Mencius* 6B14, page 75). In addition to this disparity between speech and action, the *Mencius* also considers a case of incongruity of speech and complexion. (See *Mencius* 3B7, below.)

26. See *Mencius* 3A2 (page 66).

27. See *Mencius* 6B15 (above page 65).

28. This recognition of a possibility of tampering with the connection from the heartmind to the body's periphery makes the *Mencius* seem less naive. In spite of its confidence in the principles of physiognomy, the *Mencius* gives more credence to treatment of others than to tone and visual demeanor:

> 恭者不侮人儉者不奪人
> 侮奪人之君惟恐不順焉
> 惡得為恭儉
> 恭儉豈可以聲音笑貌為哉
> Those who are respectful do not insult people.
> Those who are restrained do not rob people.
> A ruler who insults and robs people fears only that they won't obey. How could he achieve respectfulness and restraint?
> Respectfulness and restraint: how can these be obtained from tone of voice and a smiling demeanor?
> (*Mencius* 4A17)

The heartmind may tend to express itself aurally and visually, but because visual expression and tone can be manipulated, in this case, the *Mencius* values treatment of others more highly.

29. Although this is the only example of speeding horses in the *Laozi*, the *Zhuangzi* also associates hunting with pleasure and excess, like feasting:

> 夢飲酒者旦而哭泣
> 夢哭泣者旦而田獵
> 方其夢也不知其夢也
> 夢之中又占其夢焉
> 覺而後知其夢也
> One who feasts in dreams, wakes up in the morning and cries and weeps. One who cries and weeps in dreams, wakes up in the morning and goes hunting. Now, while dreaming, we do not know we are dreaming, and in the midst of a dream we can again interpret a dream. Only after waking do we know we were dreaming.
> (*Zhuangzi* 2/81)

30. The *que* 卻 is supplied from Text B.

31. An alternative possibility is suggested by Tateno Masami, who argues that the stomach may refer to the focus of meditational practice—indicating the withdrawal of consciousness during training. Tateno Masami, "A Philosophical Analysis of the Laozi from an Ontological Perspective," in *Religious and Philosophical Aspects of the Laozi,* ed. Mark Csikszentmihalyi and Philip J. Ivanhoe (Albany: State University of New York Press, 1999), 178.

32. Of course, at the political level, this also reduces the risk of revolt.

33. The following four uses of *yu* do *not* imply criticism of desire:

將欲取天下而為之
吾見其弗得已
Of those who desire to take the world and act on it—I see that they will not obtain it.
(*Laozi* 29)
(The *de yi* 得已 is supplied from Text B.)

將欲拾之必古張之
將欲弱之必古強之
If you desire to shrink it,
You must certainly stretch it.
If you desire to weaken it,
You must certainly strengthen it.
(*Laozi* 36)
(The *bi gu* 必古 is supplied from Text B.)

大邦者不過欲兼畜人
小邦者不過欲入事人
All that the large state desires is to unite and rear others; all that the small state desires is to enter and serve others.
(*Laozi* 61)

是以聖人之欲上民也
必以其言下之
其欲先民也
必以其身後之
Therefore if the sage desires to be above the people,
He must in his speech be below them.
And if he desires to be in front of the people,
He must in person be behind them.
(*Laozi* 66)
(The *min ye* 民也 is supplied from Text A.)

34. The phrase "desire not to desire" occurs again in *Laozi* 57 in the *Mawangdui* text:

> 我欲不欲而民自樸
> I desire not to desire, and the people make themselves uncarved.
> (*Laozi* 57)

It does not recur in the *Wang Bi* edition, which simply says, "I have no desires."

35. The *Wang Bi* edition has *yan* 言 for *wen*, but the *Xiang Er* edition also has *wen*.

36. The *Wang Bi* edition reads 道之出口淡乎其無味 "The way's coming out of the mouth—bland, its lack of taste!"

37. There is a concern for a rectification of standards, including compasses and squares, in the synoptic *Mozi*, the Neo-Mohist Canons, and the *Xunzi*. Given its interest in the "uncut," it is possible that the *Laozi*, like the *Zhuangzi*, objects to the cutting involved in the application of these sensory standards:

> 且夫待鉤繩
> 規矩而正者
> 是削其性者也
> Using hook and line, compass and square to make things straight, this is scraping away its *xing*.
> (*Zhuangzi* 8/13)

38. The series of accomplishments in Chapters 10 and 27 are also examples of this not completing both parts of an action:

[載]營魄抱一能無離乎
傳氣至柔能嬰兒乎
滌除元覽能無疵乎
愛民治國能無知乎
天門開闔能無雌乎
明白四達能無為乎
In regulating the *po*-spirits and embracing the one, can you do it without leaving?
In concentrating the *qi* and arriving at softness, can you be like a baby?
In cultivating and removing from the profound mirror, can you make it without blemish?
In loving the people and governing the state, can you do it without using knowledge?
When the gates of heaven open and close, can you act the female?
In clarifying the four reaches, can you do it without acting?
(*Laozi* 10, *Wang Bi* edition)

Henricks argues convincingly that the first word in line 1 belongs to the prior chapter. I take *wu* 無 in the fifth line to be *wei* 為 (Henricks, *Laozi: Te-Tao Ching*, 209).

Chapter 27 in the *Wang Bi* edition reads,

善行無轍蹟
善言無瑕謫
善數不用籌策
善閉無關楗而不可開
善結無繩約而不可解
A good walker leaves no treads behind.
A good speaker lacks flaw or fault.
A good counter does not use tallies or chips.

A good closer does not shut the bolt, yet the door cannot open.
A good tier ties without rope or cord, yet the knot cannot be untied.
(*Laozi* 27, *Wang Bi* edition)

39. The *Laozi* does express confidence in the "great image":

執大象天下往
Grasp the great image, and the world will come to you.
(*Laozi* 35)

However, the *Laozi* 41 says, "the great image lacks shape."

On the basis of parallels to other lines, the *tian* 天 in the *Mawangdui* version is probably supposed to be *da* 大.

40. The *Laozi* 14 presents a similar series of half-performed acts of discrimination.

41. In addition to the textual connections that I cite here, the use of common terms like *chu* 出 "exit" (or "emit") and *ru* 入 "enter" to describe both doors and sense discrimination also establishes a connection between them. The *Laozi*'s only use of *chu* in relation to sense discrimination refers to the *dao* coming out of the mouth (35), but other texts of the period establish the association. *Zhuangzi* 2/5 connects holes (竅 穴) with noses, mouths, eyes, and ears. *Xunzi* 25/28 implies that the ears and eyes are doors and windows. Also, the *Yu Lao* chapter of the *Han Feizi* interprets the *Laozi* 47 as saying the senses are door and windows:

空竅者神明之戶牖也
耳目竭於聲色精神竭於外貌

> Holes and cavities are the doors and windows of the *shenming* [spirit brightness?]. The ears and the eyes are exhausted by sound and color. *Jingshen* [seminal spirit?] is exhausted by outward manners.
> (*Han Feizi* 7/4)

42. In this case, the sage *does* "complete" an action, but completes without doing. This makes me hesitant to say the point is particularly aimed at not completing. Instead it seems to be a matter of doing one part of an action without the other (thereby, in some way, not "exhausting" oneself or the act).

43. The only exceptions that do not praise some form of sensory "incompleteness" are two instances of sensory knowing—knowing the whiteness (28) and knowing beautiful and ugly (2)—and two references to the *dao* being heard.

44. I take it that Hun Dun represents the human condition. By another reading, however, the drilling may have killed Hun Dun precisely because he was *not* human.

45. The nose remains open allowing breathing, which might also permit the continued interaction of *hun*-spirits during sleep.

Because the *Zhuangzi* states in a different place (1/31) that it is not just the "form and bones" (*xing hai* 形 骸) that have blindness and deafness (the heartmind has them, too), there is reason to believe that the phrase "form and bones" includes the eyes and ears (not simply the external shape). Another link suggesting that the senses in general are the part of the form that opens in this particular passage is the character *jie* 接, which is often used of the senses. See Chapter 1 note 31.

46. A less literal interpretation of *chu* 出 might read this as "manifesting"—that is, "embodying" rather than "letting out" from openings. However, *chu* is commonly used for speech being "emitted" (presumably through the mouth), although there is only one instance of this in the *Zhuangzi* itself. It says,

> 今子之所取大者先生也而猶出言若是
> 不亦過乎
> Now, the person you've selected as the most eminent is our teacher—and yet you emit speech like that? Isn't *that* also a crime?
> (*Zhuangzi* 5/18)

Along the same lines, *Zhuangzi* 2/13 says the emotions are "emitted" like music (piped through the body?) and like breath that forms mushrooms in the "hollow" between night and day.

47. The passage reads,

> 故不足以滑和不可入乎靈府
> 使之和豫通而不失於兑...
> Therefore they are not sufficient to disturb one's harmony.
> They cannot enter one's spiritual residence.
> To make it so that harmony and ease circulate, but are not lost in openings...
> (*Zhuangzi* 5/44–45)

48. Graham also translates the term as "externalize" (Graham, *Disputers of the Tao*, 198). At the risk of anachronism, it seems to mean something like the opposite of "internalize"—that is, placing something aside where it need not provoke concern. One of the *Zhuangzi*'s characters teaches another to externalize the world, things, and life itself. She says,

參日而後能外天下
已外天下矣吾又守之
七日而後能外物
已外物矣吾又守之
九日而後能外生
已外生矣而後能朝徹...
After three days, he was able to put the world outside him. When he had got the world outside him I still kept at him, and by the seventh day he was able to put things outside him. When he got things outside him, again I kept at him, and by the ninth day he was able to put life outside him. Once he had got life outside him, he could break through to a new morning...
(*Zhuangzi* 6/39–41)

49. *Laozi* 10 mentions the *po* 魄 (spirits) in the context of something not leaving, although it is not clear whether the person does not leave the *po* or vice versa.

50. *Zhuangzi* 1/31 notes that the bones and body "have blindness and deafness," hence the bones and body include the eyes and ears.

51. This indicates that roaming *outside* direction and externalizing form and bones is different from roaming *inside* direction. However, even the outside/inside distinction seems to break down, when one of the characters roams *inside* form and bones:

吾與夫子遊十九年矣
而未嘗知吾兀者也
今子與我遊於形骸之內
而子索我於形骸之外
不亦過乎

> I have been roaming with the Master for nineteen years now and never knew myself as a person with a chopped foot. Now you and I are roaming on the inside of form-and-bones, yet you haul me out to the outside of form-and-bones. Don't you think that is also a crime?
> (*Zhuangzi* 5/22–24)

The term *wai* 外 also appears once in the *Laozi*, and there too the body is externalized. However, it is done for a different purpose. The *Laozi* juxtaposes "externalize" (*wai* 外) to the term "preserve" or "survive" (*cun* 存), saying that the sage preserves his self/body precisely by "turning it out" or placing it outside of his concerns. Thus, in the *Laozi*, one actually seeks to preserve the body/self, and therefore "externalizes" it.

52. *Zhuangzi* 4/32–33 suggests that this occurs through the ears and eyes, but *Zhuangzi* 2/10 implies that the *hun* 魂 travels through the nose, as it remains open during sleep.

53. However, the "fasting of the heartmind" passage might simply state *that* they stop:

> 聽止於耳心止於符
> Listening stops at the ear. The heartmind stops at tallying.
> (*Zhuangzi* 4/27)

54. Yet, seeing does still occur, as the *jian* 見 in the following line demonstrates. After mentioning that the senses know to stop, the line continues,

> 雖然每至於族吾見其難為怵然為戒
> 視為止行為遲...

However, whenever I come to something interlocked, I *see* where it will be hard to handle and cautiously prepare myself, my looking stops, my action slows down... (*Zhuangzi* 3/10)

55. In fact, rather than promoting finding sweetness in simple foods, the *Zhuangzi* implies that sweetness has no standard and hence undermines the possibility of simple sweetness (*Zhuangzi* 2/68).

56. In contrast to the repetition of this theme in the *Zhuangzi*, only one reference to "walking without a trace" appears in the *Laozi*, in Chapter 27, which notes that someone who is good at walking leaves no tracks.

57. The heartmind measures the ear against the eye (and vice versa). Thus, in some sense, feet (now standing in for what the eye sees) serve as the standard against which speech can be tallied. The tallying of walking feet (seen by the eye) and speech (heard by the ear) seems to be what constitute knowledge.

This bears comparison to the Ode quoted in *Mencius* 5B7, in which the superior person literally *treads* a *dao*, while lower people look on. It is also related to *Mencius* 7A38, where the feet are the measure for one's words, because the sage alone is able to "tread" his shape (*xing* 形).

58. The *Zhuangzi*'s characters speak in a way that is ill-suited for measurement and correspondence:

吾聞言於接輿大而無當
I heard Jie Yu's speech—huge and not corresponding.
(*Zhuangzi* 1/27)

The *Zhuangzi*'s own words, like Hui Shi's tree, do not fit measurements:

> 惠子謂莊子曰吾有大樹人謂之樗
> 其大本擁腫而不中繩墨
> 其小枝卷曲而不中規矩立之塗
> 匠者不顧今子之言大而無用眾所同去也
>
> Said Hui Shi to Zhuangzi, "I have a great tree, people call it ailanthus. Its trunk is too squeezed and swollen to measure with an inked line, its little branches are too curly and crooked to measure with a compass or an L-square. Stand it up in the road, and a carpenter wouldn't give it a glance. Now this talk of yours is big and useless—what the masses collectively discard."
>
> (*Zhuangzi* 1/43)

References

Allan, Sarah. *The Way of Water and Sprouts of Virtue*. Albany: State University of New York Press, 1997.

Allinson, Robert E., ed. *Understanding the Chinese Mind: The Philosophical Roots*. New York: Oxford University Press, 1989.

Ames, Roger. "The Body in Classical Chinese Philosophy." In *Self as Body in Asian Theory and Practice*, edited by Thomas P. Kasulis. Albany: State University of New York Press, 1993.

Ames, Roger, ed. *Wandering at Ease in the Zhuangzi*. Albany: State University of New York Press, 1998.

Ames, Roger, and Joel Marks, eds. *Emotions in Asian Thought: A Dialogue in Comparative Philosophy*. Albany: State University of New York Press, 1995.

Ames, Roger, and Henry Rosemont, Jr. *The Analects of Confucius: A Philosophical Translation*. New York: Ballantine, 1998.

Austin, J. L. *Sense and Sensibilia*. New York: Oxford University Press, 1962.

Bockover, Mary I. "The Concept of Emotion Revisited: A Critical Synthesis of Western and Confucian Thought." In *Emotions in Asian Thought: A Dialogue in Comparative Philosophy*, 161-179. Albany: State University of New York Press, 1995.

Boltz, William G. *The Origin and Early Development of the Chinese Writing System*. New Haven: American Oriental Society, 1994.

———. "The Religious and Philosophical Significance of the 'Hsiang Erh' Lao Tzu in Light of the Ma-Wang-Tui Silk Manuscripts." *Bulletin of the School of Oriental and African Studies* 45 (1982): 95-117.

Brooks, Bruce, and Taeko Brooks. *The Original Analects: Sayings of Confucius and His Successors*. New York: Columbia University Press, 1998.

Chang, Kwang-chih. "Ancient China and its Anthropological Significance." In *Archeological Thought in America*, edited by C. C. Lamberg-Karlovsky. Cambridge: Cambridge University Press, 1989.

Chidester, David. *Word and Light: Seeing, Hearing and Religious Discourse*. Urbana, Ill.: University of Illinois Press, 1992.

Classen, Constance. *Worlds of Sense: Exploring the Senses in History and Across Cultures*. London: Routledge, 1993.

Cua, A. S. *Ethical Argumentation: A Study in Hsun Tzu's Moral Epistemology*. Honolulu: University of Hawaii Press, 1985.

Davidson, Donald. *Inquiries into Truth and Interpretation*. Oxford: Clarendon Press, 1984.

Defoort, Carine. *The Pheasant Cap Master: A Rhetorical Reading*. Albany: State University of New York Press, 1997.

Derrida, Jacques. *Writing and Difference*. Chicago: University of Chicago Press, 1978.

DeWoskin, Kenneth. *A Song for One or Two: Music and the Concept of Art in Early China*. Ann Arbor, Mich.: Center for Chinese Studies, The University of Michigan, 1982.

Elias, Norbert. "On Human Beings and Their Emotions: A Process-Sociological Essay." in *Theory, Culture, & Society* 4 (1987): 339–61.

Fingarette, Herbert. *Confucius—The Secular as Sacred.* New York: Harper and Row, 1972.

Geaney, Jane. "A Critique of A. C. Graham's Reconstruction of the 'Neo-Mohist Canons.'" *Journal of the American Oriental Society* 119.1 (1999): 1–11.

———. "Mencius's Hermeneutics." *Journal of Chinese Philosophy* 27 (2000): 93–100.

Gibbs, Donald A. "Notes on the Wind: The Term 'Feng' in Chinese Literary Criticism." In *Transition and Permanence: Chinese History and Culture*, edited by David C. Buxbaum and Frederick W. Mote. Hong Kong: Cathay Press Limited, 1972.

Goldin, Paul Rakita. *Rituals of the Way: The Philosophy of Xunzi.* Peru, Ill.: Open Court, 1999.

Graham, A. C. *Ch'uang-tzu: The Inner Chapters.* London: George Allen & Unwin, 1981.

———. *Disputers of the Tao: Philosophical Argumentation in Ancient China.* LaSalle, Ill.: Open Court, 1989.

———. *Later Mohist Logic, Ethics, and Science.* Hong Kong: Chinese University Press, 1978.

———. *Studies in Chinese Philosophy and Philosophical Literature*, Series in Chinese Philosophy and Culture. Albany: State University of New York Press, 1990.

Granet, Marcel. *La Penseé Chinoise.* Paris: Albin Michel, 1968.

Guo, Qingfan. *Zhuangzi JiShi.* Beijing: Zhongguo Shu dian ying yin, 1988.

Hall, David L., and Roger T. Ames. *Thinking through Confucius.* Albany: State University of New York Press, 1987.

Hamlyn, D. W. *Sensation and Perception*. London: Routledge and Kegan Paul, Ltd., 1961.

Han Feizi. Subu Beiyao edition. Taibei: Zhonghua Shuju, 1968.

Hansen, Chad. *A Daoist Theory of Chinese Thought*. Oxford: Oxford University Press, 1992.

———. "Language in the Heart-Mind." In *Understanding the Chinese Mind*, edited by Robert Allinson, 75–124. New York: Oxford University Press, 1989.

———. "*Qing* 情 in Pre-Buddhist Chinese Thought." In *Emotions in Asian Thought: A Dialogue in Comparative Philosophy*, edited by Joel Marks and Roger T. Ames, 181–209. Albany: State University of New York Press, 1995.

———. "Should the Ancient Masters Value Reason?" In *Chinese Texts and Philosophical Contexts: Essays Dedicated to Angus C. Graham*, edited by Henry Rosemont Jr., 179–207. LaSalle Ill.: Open Court, 1991.

Harbsmeier, Christoph. "Marginalia Sino-Logica." In *Understanding the Chinese Mind*, edited by Robert Allinson, 125–166. Hong Kong: Oxford University Press, 1989.

Harper, Donald. "Warring States Philosophy and Occult Thought." In *The Cambridge History of Ancient China: From the Origins of Civilization to 221 B.C.*, edited by Michael Loewe and Edward L. Shaughnessy,813–884. Cambridge: Cambridge University Press, 1999.

Hay, John. "The Body as Microcosmic Source." In *Self as Body in Asian Theory and Practice*, edited by Thomas P. Kasulis. Albany: State University of New York Press, 1993.

Heidegger, Martin. *Being and Time,* translated by J. Macquarrie and E. Robinson. Oxford: Basil Blackwell, 1962.

Henricks, Robert G. *Lao-Tzu Te-Tao Ching: A New Translation Based on the Recently Discovered Ma-Wang-tui Texts*. New York: Ballantine Books, 1989.

Humphrey, Nicholas. *A History of the Mind.* London: Chatto & Windus, 1992.

Ivanhoe, Philip J., and Paul Kjellberg, eds. *Essays in Skepticism, Relativism, and Ethics in the Zhuangzi.* Albany: State University of New York Press, 1996.

Jay, Martin. *Downcast Eyes.* Berkeley: University of California Press, 1993.

Keightley, David N. "Early Civilization in China." In *Heritage of China,* edited by Paul S. Ropp, 15–54. Berkeley: University of California Press, 1990.

Knoblock, John. *Xunzi: A Translation and Study of the Complete Works*. Stanford: Stanford University Press, 1994.

Kupperman, Joel. *Learning from Asian Philosophy*. Oxford: Oxford University Press, 1999.

Kuriyama, Shigehisa. "The Imagination of Winds." In *Body, Subject, and Power in China,* edited by Angela Zito and Tani Barlow, 23–41. Chicago: University of Chicago Press, 1994.

Lao, Kan. "The Early Use of the Tally in China." In *Ancient China: Studies in Early Civilization,* edited by David T. Roy and Tsuen-hsuin Tsien, 91–98. Hong Kong: Chinese University Press, 1978.

Lau, D. C. trans. *Confucius: The Analects*. New York: Penguin, 1979.

———. trans. *Lao Tzu: Tao Te Ching*. Harmondsworth, UK: Penguin Books, 1963.

———. trans. *Mencius*. Baltimore: Penguin Books, 1970.

Lau, D. C., and Roger T. Ames, trans. *Yuan Dao: Tracing Dao to Its Source*. New York: Ballantine Books, 1998.

Legge, James, trans. *The Texts of Taoism: The Tao Te Ching, The Writings of Chuang-Tzu, The Thai-Shang*. New York: Julian Press, 1959.

———. trans. *The Works of Mencius*. Oxford: Clarendon Press, 1895. Reprint, New York: Dover Publications, 1970.

Lenk, Hans, and Gregor Paul, eds. *Epistemological Issues in Classical Chinese Philosophy*. Albany: State University of New York Press, 1993.

Liao W. K., trans. *The Complete Works of Han Fei Tzu*. London: A. Probsthain, 1935–59.

Lunyu. Harvard-Yenching Institute Sinological Index Series. Reprint. Taipei: Chinese Materials and Research Aids Service Center, 1966.

Machle, Edward J. *Nature and Heaven in the Xunzi*, Series in Chinese Philosophy and Culture. Albany: State University of New York Press, 1993.

Makeham, John. *Naming and Actuality*. Albany: State University of New York Press, 1994.

Mei Y. P., trans. *The Ethical and Political Works of Mo Tse*. London: A. Probsthain, 1929.

Mengzi (Mencius). *Harvard-Yenching Institute Sinological Index Series*. Taipei: Chinese Materials and Research Aids Service Center, 1973.

Möller, Hans Georg. "The Chinese Theory of Forms and Names (*Xingming Zhi Xue*) and Its Relation to a 'Philosophy of

Signs.'" *Journal of Chinese Philosophy* 24 (1997): 179–190.

Mote, Frederick. *Intellectual Foundations of China.* New York: Alfred A. Knopf, 1971.

Mozi. Harvard-Yenching Institute Sinological Index Series. Reprint. Taipei: Chinese Materials and Research Aids Service Center, 1973.

Munro, Donald. *The Concept of Man in Early China.* Stanford: Stanford University Press, 1969.

———. ed. *Individualism and Holism: Studies in Confucian and Taoist Values.* Ann Arbor, Mich.: The University of Michigan Center for Chinese Studies, 1985.

Needham, Joseph. *Science and Civilization in China.* Cambridge: Cambridge University Press, 1954ff.

Ng, Ong-cho. "Is Emotion (*Qing*) the Source of a Confucian Antimony?" *Journal of Chinese Philosophy* 25, (1998): 169–190.

Rosemont, Henry, Jr. *Chinese Texts and Philosophical Contexts: Essays Dedicated to Angus C. Graham.* LaSalle Ill.: Open Court, 1991.

Russell, Bertrand. *The History of Western Philosophy.* New York: Simon and Schuster, 1945.

Scharfstein, Ben-Ami. "The Contextual Fallacy." In *Interpreting across Boundaries: New Essays in Comparative Philosophy*, edited by Gerald James Larson and Eliot Deutsch, 84–97. Princeton: Princeton University Press, 1988.

Shaughnessy, Edward L., and Michael Loewe, eds. *The Cambridge History of Ancient China: From the Origins of Civilization to 221 B.C.*. Cambridge: Cambridge University Press, 1999.

Sellars, Wilfred. *Empiricism and the Philosophy of Mind*. Cambridge, Mass.: Harvard University Press, 1997.

Shun, Kwong-loi. *Mencius and Early Chinese Thought*. Stanford: Stanford University Press, 1997.

Sivin, Nathan. *Medicine, Philosophy, and Religion in Ancient China*. Brookfield, VT: Variorum, 1995.

Smith, Jonathan Z. *Imagining Religion: From Babylon to Jonestown*. Chicago: University of Chicago Press, 1982.

Solomon, Robert C., "The Cross-Cultural Comparison of Emotion." In *Emotions in Asian Thought: A Dialogue in Comparative Philosophy*, 253–294. Albany: State University of New York Press, 1995.

Tateno, Masami. "A Philosophical Analysis of the Laozi from an Ontological Perspective." In *Religious and Philosophical Aspects of the Laozi*, edited by Mark Csikszentmihalyi and Philip J. Ivanhoe, 175–185. Albany: State University of New York Press, 1999.

Teiser, Stephen F. "The Spirits of Chinese Religion." In *Religions of China in Practice,* edited by Donald S. Lopez, Jr., 34–36. Princeton: University of Princeton Press, 1996.

Tu, Wei-ming. "The Continuity of Being." In *Confucianism and Ecology: The Interrelation of Heaven, Earth, and Humans,* edited by Mary Evelyn Tucker and John Berthrong, 105–22. Cambridge Mass.: Harvard University Center for the Study of World Religions, 1998.

Waley, Arthur, trans. *The Analects of Confucius*. New York: The Macmillan Company, 1938. Reprint, New York: Random House, 1989.

Wang, Tao. "Color Terms in Shang Oracle Bone Inscriptions." *Bulletin of the School of Oriental and African Studies* 59 (1996): 63–101.

Watson, Burton, trans. *Hsün Tzu: Basic Writings.* New York: Columbia University Press, 1963.

———. trans. *Mo Tzu: Basic Writings.* New York: Columbia University Press, 1963.

———. trans. *Chuang Tzu: Basic Writings.* Columbia University Press, 1964.

———. trans. *The Complete Works of Chuang Tzu.* New York: Columbia University Press, 1968.

Willard, Dallas. "Predication as Originary Violence." In *Working Through Derrida*, edited by Gary B. Madison, 120–136. Evanston, Ill.: Northwestern University Press, 1993.

Wittgenstein, Ludwig. *Philosophical Investigations,* 3rd ed., translated by G.E.M. Anscombe. New York: Macmillan, 1958.

Xu, Shen. *Shuowen jiezi* (Explanations of single component graphs and analyses of compound characters). Reprint, Beijing: Zhonghua Shuju, 1963.

Xunzi. Harvard-Yenching Institute Sinological Index Series. Reprint. Taipei: Chinese Materials and Research Aids Service Center, 1966.

Yu, Anthony. *Rereading the Stone:Desire and the Making of Fiction in* Dream of the Red Chamber. Princeton: Princeton University Press, 1997.

Zhuangzi. Harvard-Yenching Institute Sinological Index Series. Cambridge, Mass.: Harvard University Press, 1956.

Index

SOCIETY FOR ASIAN AND COMPARATIVE PHILOSOPHY
MONOGRAPH SERIES
Henry Rosemont, Jr., Editor

No. 1 *The Sage and Society: The Life and Thought of Ho Hsin-Yin*, by Ronald Dimberg, 1974

No. 2 *Studies in Comparative Aesthetics*, by Eliot Deutsch, 1975

No. 3 *Centrality and Commonality: An Essay on* Chung-Yung, by Tu Wei-Ming, 1976

No. 4 *Discourse on the Natural Theology of the Chinese,* by Gottfried W. Leibniz, translated with an introduction, notes, and commentary by Henry Rosemont, Jr., and Daniel J. Cook, 1977

No. 5 *The Logic of Gotama*, by Kisor Kumar Chakrabarti, 1978

No. 6 *Commentary on the* Lao Tzu *by Wang Pi*, translated by Ariane Rump, introduction by Wing-tsit Chan, 1979

No. 7 *Han Fei Tzu's Political Theory*, by Wang Hsiao-po and Leo S. Chang, 1986

No. 8 *The Māṇḍūkya Upaniṣad and the Agama Śāstra: An Investigation into the Meaning of the Vedānta*, by Thomas E. Wood, 1990

No. 9 *Mind Only: A Philosophical and Doctrinal Analysis of the Vijñānavāda*, by Thomas E. Wood, 1991

No. 10 *Accomplishing the Accomplished: The* Vedas *as a Source of Valid Knowledge in Śaṅkara*, by Anantanand Rambachan, 1991

No. 11 *Nāgārjunian Disputations: A Philosophical Journey through an Indian Looking-Glass*, by Thomas E. Wood, 1994

No. 12 *Ch'en Liang on Public Interest and the Law*, by Hoyt Cleveland Tillman, 1994

No. 13 *Definition and Induction: A Historical and Comparative Study,* by Kisor Kumar Chakrabarti, 1995

No. 14 *Let the Cow Wander: Modeling the Metaphors in Veda and Vedānta,* by Michael W. Myers, 1995

No. 15 *The Four Political Treatises of the Yellow Emperor: Original Mawangdui Texts with Complete English Translations and an Introduction,* by Leo S. Chang and Yu Feng, 1998

No. 16 *Perceptual Error: The Indian Theories,* by Srinivasa Rao, 1998

No. 17 *Hindu Ethics: A Philosophical Study,* by Roy W. Perrett, 1998

No. 18 *Skillful Means: The Heart of Buddhist Compassion,* by John W. Schroeder

No. 19 *On the Epistemology of the Senses in Early Chinese Thought,* by Jane Geaney

Orders should be directed to University of Hawai'i Press, 2840 Kolowalu Street, Honolulu, Hawai'i 96822. Manuscripts should be directed to Professor Henry Rosemont, Jr., Department of Philosophy, St. Mary's College, St. Mary's City, Maryland 20686.